SURVIVING BEAUTIFULLY

Your Comprehensive Guide to Aesthetic Issues
during Cancer Treatment

**VICTORIA TILLOTSON
AND
LANA KOIFMAN**

ISBN: 1499226489
ISBN 13: 9781499226485

TABLE OF CONTENTS

ACKNOWLEDGEMENTS

A PARTNERSHIP STARTS WITH TWO PEOPLE, and ends in being one. Here, we share our individual acknowledgements, as well as those we jointly celebrate.

Lana:

"You must hate your job? Knowing that you may find something terrible?" I asked the ultrasound technologist who was assisting in my biopsy. "No," she said, "I know that I am helping people learn the truth, and get the treatment they need. I am the first step on the road to survival." I never learned your name, but in my acknowledgments, it is you, Ms. Ultrasound Technologist, that I want to name first: you and every nurse and every chemo technician; every phlebotomist that gets the needle into a vein in the first try; every member of the medical team; every scientist who does the research; and every assistant who makes the appointments. You are the steps to survival. You are truly the watchers on the wall. My special thanks to the most dedicated professionals at the Memorial Sloan-Kettering Cancer Center in New York City.

There are no words to thank the doctors whose professionalism and dedication saves lives every day, and definitely saved mine. My eternal gratitude to Dr. Constantine Bakas, my OB, whose caring and compassion only equals his vigilance. Thank you to the brilliant breast surgeon, Dr. Karen Arthur, who promised that something good will come out of this ordeal. I hope that Surviving Beautifully is just part of that "something." My oncology team was headed by the truly gifted Dr. Diana Lake. Because of her confidence and kindness, I knew that I was getting the best care in the world. Every week, we spoke about our teenage kids, and I sincerely hope that her son knows that his mother makes a real difference EVERY DAY.

The project Surviving Beautifully was born from a meeting of minds in a coffee shop in Armonk, but the idea was born in the office of Dr. Danielle Deluca-Pytell, my plastic reconstruction surgeon. It was here when I first felt hope of not only getting through this ordeal, but that I had a chance of getting back to old self. I stopped being just a patient and again became a woman. Every time I look at myself in the mirror, I thank God for the talent He has given Dr. Deluca-Pytell. Thank you to Dr. Anca Tchelebi-Moscatello and her staff at Park Avenue Medical Spa in Armonk for helping me take care of my skin during my treatments. Dr. Tchelebi believed in the project of Surviving Beautifully from its very inception because she knows how critical self image is to a woman.

I believe in time of crisis, an angel comes. My angel is Lena Armel, a beautiful survivor. She came to have lunch with me before every one of my treatments. Enough said.

Thank you to my daughters, Renee and Megan. To Renee, thank you for all the ideas, support, work and enthusiasm that you put into helping us with this book and this project. To both of them, thank you for existing and for reminding me every day that life is worth fighting for.

You do not have to be related by blood to be family, but rather have your souls connect. You can be born in another country, on another continent and in a different hemisphere and still be my soul sister, Edith Cobos. When I was in trouble, I called you first. I always do, and you always come.

Last, because it is most important, all my love and gratitude to my husband, Igor, who made me feel beautiful even on the ugliest days.

Victoria:

I am fortunate to not have experienced cancer firsthand. Cancer was in fact the farthest thing from my mind when Lana approached me about Surviving Beautifully. The very idea of writing about cancer, much less cancer and beauty, seemed odd indeed.

However, soon after my mother was dying of a cancer-related illness. She agonized over her looks, her thinning hair, her inability to wear what she wanted. She felt helpless and alone with these concerns. It dawned on me that she could benefit from this project. My mother died before being able to see this book, but I know she would have been proud. It is her memory that I dedicate it.

I would like to give special thanks to my husband, David, who has stood shoulder to shoulder with me from day one. I simply could not have written this book without him, and Surviving Beautifully is better for having him here with us.

I also wish to thank my sister Emma St. Germain, RN, for her never-ending emotional support, and practical assistance with foreign and intimidating medical information, to my dear friends Heidi Macalle, Peggy and Ed Strauss, Liz Dalton, Sarah and Rob Schmieder, and Diane Jones, and to Kristen McVeety, for always being there to help with the nuts-and-bolts legal stuff involved in our project. I would also like to thank Leo Guthart for his continued support.

Us:

Throughout this project we have sought to never doubt that we would make Surviving Beautifully happen…and make it a success. We are profoundly grateful to those who felt the same way; who provided us expert information, insight as survivors, business advice, or just propped up our spirits, and egos, when we were daunted and confused.

We are particularly thankful to early supporters who were able to feel our passion and see the importance of Surviving Beautifully while we stumbled along the uncharted paths to its realization: to Sharon Bowers, Victoria's literary agent who never wavered from her belief that Surviving Beautifully was a great idea and should be published; to skin care expert Anne C. Willis, who "got it" immediately even when we struggled to explain our project in a loud and crowded restaurant in the heart of Chelsea; to C. Andrew Salzberg, MD, a true pioneer in the area of reconstructive surgery, and the first of our experts to come aboard; to comedian and survivor Jenny Saldaña, who shared her expertise, contacts, unabashed joy and humor with us over lunch and in Bryant Park; to Jodie Guerrero, our comrade in arms in Australia who is the very definition of a beautiful survivor; to our web designer Oliver Christie, who calmly but firmly us onto the Internet; to our dear friend and stylist extraordinaire Colin Megaro; and to makeup artist Tim Quinn who, despite his indescribably busy schedule of fashion shoots and runway shows, responded to each and every one of Victoria's emails. Thank you.

INTRODUCTION

by Lana Koifman

THE IDEA FOR THIS BOOK WAS born on a Friday afternoon while I sat on the floor of my home office loudly sobbing into the telephone to my best friend, "I cannot take it anymore! When is it going to stop?" This was not the day of I heard my diagnosis, but already a month after my chemo treatments when my hair was still falling out. Because I was part of the study group at Memorial Sloan-Kettering Cancer Center and my treatments were new, my oncologist was not able to tell me the full extent of my side effects. The "side effects" of my lifesaving treatments, my mastectomy and my reconstructive surgeries, and my hair thinning stopped being "side" anything and became the center of my life. They were significantly eroding my self confidence and my body image.

Anyone who tells you that a big scar is a small price to pay has never paid that price. Physical and aesthetic effects of cancer treatments are as real and can be as devastating as the disease itself. It took me a lot of research and trials, but I realized that as survivors we are not powerless. Just as bravely as you battle cancer, you can proactively and successfully battle the physical side effects. You can wake up in the morning and be happy with what you see in the mirror.

When people ask my age, I often want to say that I am six years old or, rather, that my new life has existed for six years. I have been a survivor of breast cancer for that long. I was diagnosed on December 7, 2007, four days after my forty-first birthday. This date has changed me more than any other date in my life. During these past six years, I have suffered more and rejoiced more; I was the closest to dying and have lived more than ever before. I used to hate the word *survivor* because it seemed very passive, as though a person just allowed things to happen to her and got through it. When I became a survivor myself, I realized that surviving and living your own way was the *bravest* thing you could do. To survive beautifully—to emerge from grief, from pain, from loss; to take control of your own identity; to retain dignity; and to be happy with what you see in the mirror—is the most proactive thing you can do.

Before December 7, 2007, I was living the American dream. When I was nine, I immigrated with my parents to the United States from Ukraine. While my parents worked hard, I studied diligently and entered Fordham University on a full scholarship. I graduated magna cum laude, worked at Ernst & Young, married my high school sweetheart, and had two children. In 1995 my husband and I quit our jobs to start a CPA practice. I was a mother, a wife, and a successful businesswoman. I lived the life I wanted—a full, active life taking care of myself and my family. The words no woman wants to hear interrupted my American dream: "I am so sorry, but you have breast cancer."

One out of eight women in the United States will hear those words in her lifetime, and almost 40 percent of all Americans will face a fight with some type of cancer in their lives. However, hearing those words made me feel like the loneliest person in the world. I was awash with grief, disbelief, and, most importantly, *fear*. "I have just left the land of the living and entered the land of the sick," I thought to myself. I knew that I would have to go through painful surgeries (which I did, four of them) and debilitating treatments, but that was not what I feared the most. I was scared that even if I survived it all, I would never recover myself—*my self*. I worried that my sense of self would forever be lost to me, that I would never be able to look in the mirror and not see damaged goods. I was concerned about others too. What would seeing me bald and looking ill do to my parents? What would it do to my marriage? Would my husband only look at me and my destroyed breast with pity? Would my clients lose confidence in me if they thought that I was sick?

After the first long hours of complete sorrow, I realized that the only way I could get through this was to take a proactive approach to my health and my life. Even though my life would not be the same, I still needed to live *a life.* Visits to the doctor and treatments would have to be priorities, but they could not be the only things in my life. I could not afford them to be. I needed to go to work, to my children's school, and to social events. I wanted to understand how my treatments would proceed and how my appearance would change so I could make plans. My medical condition was taking so much away from me; retaining even a little control became crucial. Finally, and probably most importantly, I had to find hope.

Illness and *cancer* are words people do not typically associate with beauty. In fact, cancer and its treatments not only wreak havoc and devastation on a victim's body and emotional well-being, but they can destroy a woman's feelings of femininity and her sense of self. When battling a life-threatening illness like cancer, most women are advised about treatments, surgeries to undergo, medications to take, and support to seek. Doctors and health-care providers tend to be the most concerned with helping patients heal. However, while modern women fight to survive, they also live in the real world of boardrooms and PTA meetings, celebrations and milestones, families and colleagues—occasions and people that demand attention despite how they feel and regardless of how they look.

When I was healing, I wanted information—contemporary, sophisticated information on how to take care of myself and my appearance during my treatments. I had simple questions ("Can I use a self-tanner to brighten my complexion?") and more complex ones ("What will my breast look like after the expander is fully inflated?"). My husband was having a high school reunion, and I needed to understand what kind of a dress I could buy. My tax season was coming up, and I had to meet with a multitude of clients every day. I never dreamed that information would be so difficult to obtain. I was surprised to learn that oncologists do not know how to deal with aesthetic issues. However, I could not blame them. They are incredibly busy trying to save people's lives. Even when they learned information from patients who were able to gather it on random basis, they did not keep notes. Only a few dermatologists had specific knowledge about issues faced by people undergoing cancer treatments.

Despite spending hours every night searching the Internet and reading books, I was frustrated to find little to help me. Plenty of articles provided generic information, such as "Be gentle to your skin; do not use abrasive washes." The books dealing with beauty and cancer either concentrated on makeup application or were written well before lasers and treatments like microdermabrasion were even invented. Of course, doctors had written some excellent books about reconstruction, but I did not have the time or emotional energy to learn medical terms. Every night I read blogs and comments by women just like me asking questions and begging for practical, up-to-date information that would help them deal with physical changes during their treatments and enable them to restore themselves after the treatments were done. It was terrible draining.

Surviving Beautifully was born of this frustration, of this learn-as-you-go approach, of the mistakes I made along the way...and the triumphs too. It contains the most up-to-date and sophisticated information on all aspects of aesthetic concerns, care, and solutions of triumphing over cancer beauti-fully. This book benefits not only the patient but her doctors and health-care providers in the medical community. The conversations that commonly take place in the waiting rooms among female cancer patients are not always the ones of a medical nature that take place in examination rooms, but are of equal importance and must be addressed. Indeed, medical professionals often are not aware of the latest beauty technology that their patients may use or wish to explore. To that end, *Surviving Beautifully* provides medical professionals with a comprehensive, sophisticated, and readily available source of information to pass along to empower and educate their patients... and themselves. Thus we see *Surviving Beautifully* as a reference book and office staple for oncologists, plastic surgeons, social workers, and nurses to truly help *them* help their cancer patients during their healing journeys. Caregivers, relatives, and friends will also benefit from the information pre-sented to enhance their knowledge of how to comfort their loved ones dur-ing their healing and to help them make the choices that are right for them. When going through my healing process, and in the days that followed, I always reminded myself of the profound words of psychologist Viktor

Frankl: "Everything can be taken away from a man, but one thing: the last of the human freedoms—to choose one's attitude in any given set of circumstances, to choose one's own way."

This book is a comprehensive reference guide to let you know what to expect and how best to proceed. It addresses both the most basic and the most complex beauty and body issues during cancer treatment. This book will also help you when your treatments are over. The stress of fighting can damage skin, nails, and hair, but both at-home cures and sophisticated doctor's-office-only techniques can bring out the most beautiful you. A wonderful actress, Helen Mirren, made a very powerful statement when she said, "The way we look is part of our human condition. It is tribal, social, and personal. I don't think it's superficial; it's quite profound." This book is a tool to help you take a proactive approach to your healing, both physically and in your soul.

Please note: The information in *Surviving Beautifully* comes from experts in their fields. However, please always check with your medical team before trying products, procedures and tips from this book.

CHAPTER ONE

SKIN CARE DURING CANCER TREATMENT

ON THE FIRST DAY OF CHEMOTHERAPY, I was sitting in the waiting room at the Evelyn H. Lauder Breast Center at Memorial Sloan Kettering. I dressed carefully, just as I always do to face challenges and "enemies" such as job interviews, unpleasant conversations, and speaking engagements. An attractive blonde of "uncertain age" sat next to me. She looked me over and said unceremoniously, "Did they warn you that you cannot use Botox or do any lasers during chemo?" *No*, they did not tell me anything. As a matter of fact, the people on my oncology team (as awesome as they were) had a lot of trouble answering questions about skin care. Could I use my favorite cream with a touch of retinoid? Could I wear a self-tanner? Could I still get facials?

I realized then that fighting cancer not only meant spending endless hours in doctors' offices, but also a change in my grooming routine and beauty rituals. Cancer treatments can cause many changes in skin appearance: dry skin, redness, and acne to more serious skin conditions that board-certified dermatologists must monitor and treat. You will have to avoid many familiar cosmetic ingredients and postpone several modern antiaging treatments.

Whether you are a three-hundred-dollar facial cream consumer or soap-and-water kind of woman, this may be the time to rethink the way to care for your skin. However, you will not have to put up with looking dehydrated, sallow, or aged. As in any other chapter in this book, we will provide you with choices for taking care of yourself and your skin.

Your skin speaks volumes about your health. Never ignore changes in skin appearance because they may alert your oncology team to other serious conditions. This is not the time for wait-and-see tactics. Make a board-certified dermatologist part of your team. Involving a board-certified dermatologist in your cancer treatment can help you get through the dark times and help give you a sense of having control.

If you have never done more than wash your face in the morning and at night, you may find that using a moisturizer is very important. Wonderful, natural, "from your kitchen" recipes for soothing facials and masks can leave skin feeling and looking healthier. We will explain the importance of sun block and how to keep your regimen effective and time efficient.

Many sophisticated approaches you can take will guarantee that you emerge from your cancer journey without additional wrinkles, skin discoloration, and other signs of aging. This chapter will speak about preparing your skin prior to beginning cancer treatments, adjusting beauty regimens to include milder yet effective products, and restoring your skin after chemotherapy and radiation.

Cancer does enough damage without allowing it to diminish your self-image and rob you of confidence. As with anything

> **THE EMOTIONAL COST OF SKIN ISSUES.**
>
> *"Skin changes are a frequently reported side-effect of cancer treatment, especially with radiotherapy. Research on the psychological effects of skin irritations during treatment is a very new area…patients report that skin changes cause physical discomfort, emotional distress, altered body image, and interfere with daily functioning and life quality. Women self-medicate, use complementary therapies and psychological coping strategies to deal with these effects… Skin changes may reveal one's status as a cancer survivor before one is ready to do so. From a clinical point of view, educating patients in advance about what to expect, giving them an opportunity to express their concerns, and doing cognitive restructuring to help them base their self-worth more."*
>
> —Melanie Greenberg, Ph.D.

else, you need information and weapons to wage the best battle. Specific skin care product suggestions can be found in our Appendix.

In this chapter, we will discuss the following:

- Commonly experienced skin issues
- Caring for skin during cancer treatment
- Ingredients to avoid
- Spa treatments
- Skin treatments after the healing
- Skin care for women of color
- Nail care during cancer treatment

YOUR SKIN DURING CHEMOTHERAPY, RADIATION, AND OTHER CANCER THERAPIES

In general, chemo, radiation, and other cancer treatments reduce the skin to its raw state, and therefore may require a change in your skin care. Previously hardy skin may now be fragile and sensitive to favorite products. You may not be able to tolerate the smell of products used formerly—and that can include such items like toilet paper and laundry detergent. And sometimes your skin can suddenly have acne.

SIDE EFFECTS OF CHEMOTHERAPY ON THE SKIN

Chemotherapy treats cancer with certain chemicals that are usually poisonous to cells (cytotoxic) and therefore kill off cancer cells. According to the American Cancer Society, more than one hundred chemotherapy drugs are used in various combinations, each of which is called a chemotherapy "cocktail." The benefit of using

> **CHEMO AND SKIN 101.**
> *"Chemotherapeutic agents often target quickly dividing cells, and skin is full of them. This means that skin reactions are common with chemotherapy. Also, as our largest organ, the skin can develop intensely inflamed...as a reaction to the stresses the body in enduring with chemotherapy."*
> —Dr. Noëlle Sherber, *board-certified dermatologist*

more than one drug for cancer treatment is that it reduces the risk of your body becoming resistant to the drug; the negative is that you experience side effects in multiples because each drug brings about its own set of side effects and chemo affects *all* the body's cells. Please view our chemotherapy chart in the Appendix.

Chemotherapy can interfere with your skin's normal functioning in many ways. Here is what you might experience:

- You may have dry and scratchy eyes, dry mouth, and vaginal dryness.
- Your skin may be thin and lose elasticity, causing brittleness and irritation.
- Skin may become more reactive to sunlight (photosensitive). This condition can cause even dark-skinned women to get sunburn-like symptoms.
- Adult acne and rashes from oil overproduction may develop. Epidermal growth factor receptors (EGFRs) in particular can bring on an acne-like rash that appears about a week to ten days after treatment begins.
- Nails may exhibit discoloration, thinning, brittleness, and malformation (see information on nail care at end of this chapter).
- Menopausal symptoms may emerge from suppressing the ovaries' production of estrogen. Symptoms include dryness, hot flashes, night sweats, changes in skin texture, and accelerated signs of aging. Selective estrogen-receptor modulators (SERMs) can cause this. See our chemotherapy chart in the Appendix.
- Hand-foot syndrome (acral erythema/palmar-plantar erythrodysesthesia) can develop. See below.
- Acne, rosacea, eczema, psoriasis, fungal infections, and even herpes can become worse.
- Wounds may take longer to heal, and you may be more prone to infection.

SIDE EFFECTS OF RADIATION ON THE SKIN

Radiation therapy uses ionizing radiation by a beam (or beams) aimed at a cancerous tumor to kill cancerous cells by damaging its DNA. It is considered a "local" cancer treatment, and as such usually has fewer side effects than chemotherapy. Radiation beams are now extremely accurate. However, they also need to be aimed at the area surrounding the tumor from several angles to make sure it is completely covered if the patient moves during treatment, and to reduce chances of recurrence. Therefore, radiation can damage healthy surrounding skin as well as cancerous tissue, and may affect a large area of skin.

"Because chemotherapy attacks the rapidly dividing healthy cells in the skin at the same time that it is destroying cancerous cells, it is vital to treat your skin with the focus on protection, hydration and soothing rather than exfoliating and promoting more cell turnover."
—Dr. Anca Tchelebi-Moscatello, founder of Park Avenue Medical Spa

In breast cancer treatment, radiation may be accompanied by the draining of lymph nodes if doctors determine they are involved in the tumor. Radiation may be used before surgery, after surgery, or in conjunction with surgery and chemotherapy (radio-chemotherapy).

Although radiation may produce fewer side effects than can chemotherapy, it can affect the skin in unpleasant and sometimes painful ways due to the damage caused by the radiation to the rapidly dividing cells around the area of treatment. It usually takes the form of irritation and peeling but can sometimes be much worse. And very rarely, radiation can even bring on skin cancer.

Radiation side effects at the area of treatment can include the following:

- Reddened skin as if sunburned, then extremely dry, itchy, and irritated at the area of treatment
- A blistery rash (moist desquamation) that occurs in the fold beneath the breast or between the breast and the arm if you have radiation for breast cancer
- Skin fissures and breaks
- Skin darkening at the site of treatment, sometimes permanently

- Darkened freckles or moles
- Increased photosensitivity and with it, increased risk of skin cancer (which makes it very important to stay out of the sun while undergoing radiation treatment and for a few months afterward)
- Charring to the skin, exposing the raw subdermis
- "Wet action": oozing, blistering, and peeling
- Broken capillaries around site of radiation

Skin reactions typically start two to three weeks into treatment and subside about three to four weeks after treatment ends. However, some permanent reminders may remain in the form of darkened skin, particularly at the breast fold if you have had radiation.

OTHER CANCER TREATMENTS

A common procedure for screening and treating skin cancer is Mohs surgery (chemosurgery). In this technique, a dermatologist removes skin on and around the suspect area layer by layer with minimal damage to healthy issue around the area. At the same time, a pathologist examines each layer for cancerous cells as it is removed and while the patient waits. The pathologist then tells the surgeon where to remove tissue next. Mohs is most often performed with basal cell carcinoma, the most common form of skin cancer. This methodic technique allows the surgeon to precisely remove the cancerous tissue, preserving a larger area of healthy tissue. It also offers a high cure rate (up to 99 percent).

Although most people heal easily from this minimally invasive procedure, occasionally a patient will need a skin graft or flap if the area is large, or the surgeon may close the incision for a plastic surgeon to repair at a later time.

For many women, the procedure causes few side effects to the skin. However, some side effects may come about:

- Darkening at the area of treatment
- Raised (keloid) scar
- Numbness at area of treatment
- Skin graft resulting in change of texture

ENDOCRINE AND HORMONE THERAPY AND TAMOXIFEN

In some cases, removing estrogen that the ovaries produce improves the outcome of breast and other cancers. This is often accomplished through endocrine therapy drugs such as aromatase inhibitors that prevent the last stage of estrogen production and the additive therapy drugs that block estrogen from interacting with the estrogen receptors in cancer cells, the most common of which is tamoxifen. Generally, these therapies have less impact on the skin than chemotherapy cocktails.

These are things you may experience:

- Severely dry skin that has lost its elasticity
- Increased wrinkling, aging, and sallowness
- Skin prone to infection and wounds taking longer to heal
- Bruising
- Rashes and other irritation
- Hot flashes and acne
- Sunburn or sunburn-like symptoms

MORE SERIOUS SIDE EFFECTS

- Occasionally, a skin condition experienced during cancer treatment may be severe and indicate other medical issues. Be mindful of your skin, and if you suspect your skin issues are more than just irritation from the treatments, contact your oncology team immediately. Here are some things to look out for, keeping in mind that *early detection of symptoms aids in the cure.*
- *Neuropathy*: numbness, burning pain, loss of sensation in hands and feet, and clumsiness. These could be signs of chemotherapy-induced peripheral neuropathy (CIPN), a disorder caused by nerve damage from injury, infection, metabolic problems, and toxin exposure from chemotherapy.

- *Hives*: red, itchy welts on the surface called urticaria. While it is not common, it is caused by an allergic reaction to chemotherapy drugs, often L-asparaginase, paclitaxel, docetaxel, teniposide, procarbazine, and cytarabine. See your doctor immediately; a severe allergic reaction can be anaphylactic, which can cause shock and occasionally death.

- *Swelling*: swelling on tongue, mouth, and lips (angioedema). Another allergic reaction to chemotherapy drugs, which may become dangerous if swelling causes difficulty in breathing.

- *Skin lesions or ulcers*: scaly, inflamed skin lesions and open ulcers, sometimes accompanied by rash. This could be subacute cutaneous lupus erythematosus (SCLE). It may be a symptom of anemia as well as a reaction either to chemotherapy or UV radiation. See your doctor.

- *Hand-foot syndrome*: See "Frequently Asked Questions about Skin Care."

FINDING THE RIGHT DERMATOLOGIST

Although these side effects may sound scary, the right dermatologist can really help. In fact, we recommend you make a dermatologist part of your oncology team. Here are some tips to find the best one for you:

- *Ask the people on your oncology team if they know a dermatologist with whom they have worked in the past. This will make communication among the specialists much easier and may help treatment move more quickly.*
- *Make sure the dermatologist is board certified. Check with the American Academy of Dermatology (www.aad.org) and American Society for Dermatologic Surgery (www.asds.net).*
- *Ask if he or she has experience with oncology patients and what special precautions takes when treating them.*
- *Consider the dermatologist's office location. Your cancer treatments may make you more tired than usual, so find a doctor who se office is close and convenient.*
- *Check out any prospective doctor's website. Look for credentials, areas of specialty, and services. The site itself can indicate a lot: while it does not need to be fancy, slick, or complicated, it should be professional.*
- *Make sure you are comfortable with the doctor. If he or she belittles your concerns about skin or beauty in general, is insensitive to the fact that you're undergoing chemotherapy or radiation, or otherwise makes you uncomfortable, politely leave.*

- *New skin growth or change in a mole*: can be an indication of skin cancer itself. See our sidebar below about the importance of self-examination, and see your doctor immediately if a new growth or visible changes.

THE WARNING SIGNS OF SKIN CANCER.

The major culprit of skin cancer—the number one cancer in the United States—is excessive sun exposure. It is almost always curable when detected early and is preventable by limiting sun exposure and using sunscreen. Most skin cancers form in older people on parts of the body exposed to the sun or in people who have weakened immune systems. However, radiation as part of treatment for another cancer can also be a risk factor in non-melanoma cancers. Like any other cancer, early detection is paramount. Make a yearly dermatology appointment for a full body check, and do a self-examination once a month.

According to the National Cancer Institute, skin cancer typically has four forms:

- *Melanoma: skin cancer that forms in melanocytes (skin cells that make pigment). Melanoma is the most dangerous of skin cancers, as it can metastasize quickly to other parts of the body. It can reveal itself as an existing mole that has changed in shape, color, or size; it can also start as a new spot.*
- *Basal cell carcinoma: skin cancer that forms in the lower part of the epidermis (the outer layer of the skin). This usually shows up as an uncolored mole or a pimple that just won't heal.*
- *Squamous cell carcinoma: skin cancer that forms in squamous cells (flat cells that form the surface of the skin). This typically manifests as a crusty or scaly patch of skin that won't respond to a skin treatment.*
- *Merkel cell carcinoma, or MCC: skin cancer that forms in neuroendocrine cells (cells that release hormones in response to signals from the nervous system). It is mostly found in Caucasian skin. While MCC does not have a specific sign, it usually manifests as a painless, firm, flesh-colored to red or blue bump that sometimes grows quite quickly.*

Warning signs include the following:

- *A skin growth that increases in size and appears pearly, translucent, tan, brown, black, or multicolored*
- *A mole, birthmark, beauty mark, or any brown spot that changes color, increases in size or thickness, changes in texture, is irregular in outline, is bigger than 6 mm or a quarter inch (the size of a pencil eraser), or appears after age twenty-one*
- *A spot or sore that continues to itch, hurt, crust, scab, erode, or bleed*
- *An open sore that does not heal within three weeks*

The use of sunscreen is a *critical step* you should take at every point in your life. In his book *Age-Less*, Dr. Fredric Brandt states: "Everyone needs to consider sun block as vital as toothpaste...research has shown that 40 percent to 50 percent of Americans who live to age sixty-five will have skin cancer at least once." You don't want to survive one bout of chemotherapy only to have to go through it again, so load up on sun protection every day, no matter what you are doing and whether you will be indoors or out.]

HOW TO PREPARE YOUR SKIN FOR CANCER TREATMENT

Many different ways to approach skin care during cancer treatment are available, but experts from many different fields concur on one basic principal: *protect, hydrate, and soothe the skin as much as possible.* Chemotherapy thins the skin and makes it prone to infection and irritation; radiation can irritate the skin and cause it to open, inviting infection as well. To help skin perform its protective function, you must do things to strengthen it and restore what has been compromised by the chemotherapy treatment.

This is not the time to experiment with aggressive new procedures, treatments, or formulations unless under medical care. You also should not be using products that strip the skin of moisture and oil or encourage the overturn of cells through dermabrasion or other aggressive exfoliating techniques. And finally, be sure to clear *all* products and procedures with your oncology team before use.

What to Look for in Products

Before and during treatment, consider using products that are:

- Fragrance-free
- Created for sensitive or compromised skin
- Devoid of the chemicals listed in our "danger zone" section below
- Free from mineral oil, petroleum, or other heavy oils that can clog pores; while this is a personal choice, many dermatologists agree on this
- Formulations with minimal synthetic ingredients
- Baby products

Avoid products that do any of the following:

- Compromise the skin's barrier through cell turnover, such as retinoids or rough scrubs. Not only will they irritate your skin and sometimes cause a painful rash, they may create microscopic cuts that take a long time to heal. (On occasion, a light scrub may be OK; see below.)
- Contain any kind of abrasive, acidic, or alkaline ingredients, including fruit acids
- Contain fragrances, alcohol, detergents, or colors.
- Contain the following ingredients:
  1. Benzoyl peroxide and other topical acne preparations (unless approved by your doctor)
  2. Astringents and other drying agents
  3. Metals often found in skin-care products containing alpha and beta hydroxy acids or other peeling agents
  4. Botanical ingredients that may cause irritation such as arnica, ginseng, menthol, tea tree, camphor, eucalyptus, and wintergreen
  5. Unpreserved products that may cause contamination or infection; naturally preserved products are usually fine
  6. Abrasive cleansing devices like loofahs and pumice stones

HELP YOUR HOME ENVIRONMENT TO SUPPORT SKIN HEALTH

Your environment and habits are important to consider in terms of your skin care during cancer treatment. While you are not in control of toxins, fumes, or other irritants in

> **BABY YOUR SKIN.**
> *"I talk with my patients who are undergoing breast cancer treatment about the importance of babying their skin, literally! Baby skin care products are often a good choice since they tend to be mild, moisturizing, and free from a lot of synthetic fragrance. While undergoing cancer treatment, many patients will notice a heightened or altered sense of smell that will make them want to avoid a lot of synthetically fragranced products."*
> —Dr. Noëlle Sherber

the air outside, you are fully capable of making your home as supportive to your health as possible. You can do several things in your house to aid skin care during your treatment.

- Use a humidifier to add moisture to the air. In her book *Heal Your Skin*, Dr. Ava Shamban suggests that air moisture is important "particularly in the bedroom while you sleep... Be sure to choose [a humidifier] with cool or adjustable capabilities, a good filter, and a UV-antimicrobial feature so as not to spread airborne viruses, bacteria, and molds." She likes the VicksV3800 Cool Mist Tower Humidifier and Germ Guardian H-30000 Ultrasonic Humidifier.
- Use fragrance-free laundry detergent, dryer sheets, toilet paper, facial tissue, and household cleansers that may come in contact with skin. If you have a housekeeper or housecleaning service, be sure to provide them with the products you wish to use so they don't use harsh, heavily scented industrial-strength cleaners.
- Remove scented candles and discontinue using air fresheners.
- Use two kinds of gloves for household chores: rubber or latex gloves for dishes and chores like washing the dog, watering the garden, and scrubbing the floor. Complement these with thin, unbleached cotton gloves for dusting, organizing, vacuuming, etc. Be sure to clean the latex gloves often to avoid bacteria.
- Avoid spray-on dusting products and use a damp microfiber towel or Swiffer-type duster.
- Do not feel embarrassed if you feel safer wearing a mask while doing chores: disposable paper masks are readily available in surgical supply stores.
- If you suspect your house has asbestos or mold, now is a good time to double-check.

HOW TO HANDLE YOUR SKIN DURING TREATMENT

Before we talk about what specific products you can safely use on your skin, let's talk a little about how to care for your skin. Even the most benign skin-care products can be harmful if used incorrectly or aggressively.

- Use a light touch when cleansing, drying and applying products
- Avoid aggressively wiping the skin.
- After bathing, pat your skin dry with a soft, freshly laundered towel each time. Do not rub! A microfiber towel may be a good choice, as it absorbs more water than a traditional terrycloth one and reduces the need to rub.
- Avoid long soaks in the bath and hot showers, which can dry skin and also open pores, inviting infection. Similarly, avoid steam rooms and saunas.
- Get in the habit of *pressing* products into the skin rather than slathering vigorously.
- Use disposable sponges/cloths and cotton rounds rather than washcloths, which can remain damp and breed bacteria. Resist the temptation to reuse sponges and cosmetic wedges.
- Make sure you are the only one using your skin products during treatment! You want to avoid exposing your skin to bacteria as much as possible.
- Use little spoons or plastic spatulas to remove products from their containers,

YOUR NEW ROUTINE DURING TREATMENT

No matter what you have done in the past, doctors agree that your skin routine should now be based on the CPHS approach (cleanse, protect, hydrate, and soothe). This means hands and lips too. Here are the basics from Dr. Cynthia Bailey.

> *"The most important message I would like to send out about skin care is no matter what the regimen is, whether expensive or frugal, from the drugstore or out-of-the-kitchen, it must be consistent. It is crucial to learn to be good to yourself; to take care of yourself; and to make yourself your own project."*
> —*Lana Koifman*

Cleanse

- Use only gentle cleansers. Your skin is protected from chapping by an outer dead skin cell layer called the stratum corneum. The foaming agent in many soaps remove your natural lipids (oils) that hold this layer together, causing it to weaken. When you take that weakened layer out into the world it can't hold up. Switch your cleansers right now to support your fragile skin.

- Use a gentle cleanser *and only where you need it.* This means parts of your skin that have the body odor glands, including your armpits, groin, buttocks, and feet. If you have oily skin, use cleanser on the oily areas of your back, neck, and chest

- For your face, use the mildest cleanser that does the job. Don't shoot for that tight "squeaky clean" feeling after washing. This actually means that you removed too much of your natural oils and irritated your skin. If your skin is excessively flaky and not sensitive, you can carefully try a very gentle exfoliating scrub.

- To avoid drying out your hands, use cleanser only on your palms most of the time. The skin on the back of your hand is much more fragile and prone to dryness. Also, rinse all the cleanser out from between your fingers where "dishpan hands" usually starts because of retained soap residue.

- If you are very dry, opt for a surfactant-free (detergent- or soap-free) cleanser that you tissue, rather than rinse, off. These cleansers preserve the skin's moisture level and also build up a protective layer because they sit on the skin. Cetaphil and La Roche-Posay Toleriane Dermo-Cleanser are two examples of surfactant-free cleansers.

- Sometimes cancer treatments will actually cause oily skin. "Oily/acne prone skin is best treated with cleansers that contain salicylic acid, which is a lipid soluble acid that helps clean pores out, topical antibiotics such as benzoyl peroxide or clindamycin as well as a solution or gel with salicylic acid or a retinoid which will do the same thing," says Dr. Fredric Brandt.

Protect

- Keep skin hydrated with a hydrophilic, protective moisturizer that also soothes itching (including skin on the body). Moisturize religiously to slow down the skin's loss of water. Keeping skin moist will make you more comfortable and plump up the skin to make it look fresher.
- Use broad-spectrum, non-chemical sunscreen (meaning it contains titanium dioxide or zinc oxide that creates a physical barrier on the skin) with a minimum SPF of 30. A sunscreen for babies that is unscented may be a good choice.

Hydrate and Soothe

Moisturize with richly hydrating skin moisturizers immediately after washing any part of your skin. Moisturizers only work if they are applied right after you've had your skin in water because they trap the water that you just soaked up into your skin. For example, moisturize the following at these times:

- Body: right after your bath or shower
- Face: morning and night
- Hands: many times during the day, whenever you wash or feel dry
- Lips: coat them throughout the day with a hydrating lip balm, especially when you're outdoors or in hot, dry, indoor air. Aquaphor is a favorite of dermatologists.

Please see our suggestions for skin care products in the Appendix.

> *"Lips may become cracked and dry with chemotherapy. But a dermatologist should check that there isn't a yeast infection, called perleche. For perleche, a prescription anti-yeast anti-inflammatory ointment called Mycolog works wonders and, in a pinch, over-the-counter Nystatin cream can be mixed into Aquaphor."*
> —*Dr. Noëlle Sherber*

HOMEMADE MASKS

During healing, you may wish to take a natural approach to skin care, and one way to do it is by using homemade masks that focus on gentle cleansing, soothing and treatment. A popular aesthetician at Park Avenue Medical Spa shared these masks from her native country of Poland. She adds: "Sensitive skin should be treated with very gentle products. When using the natural facial masks, consider that the lemon juice can increase the sensitivity of the skin while chamomile, oatmeal, yogurt, or avocado have a calming effect. Thus, use these ingredients accordingly."

Tips for Homemade Masks:

- Unless otherwise noted, keep the mask on for about ten minutes and wash off with tepid water.
- Use masks in the evening. Your skin will absorb the ingredients more easily overnight.
- Apply moisturizer after washing the mask off.
- Use common sense when mixing the ingredients unless the exact amount is specified. The mask's consistency should be such that it will not slide off the face.
- These masks can be used two to three times a week. If you find them particularly soothing and enjoyable, you can alternate masks and do one every day.

Cleansing Masks

All-purpose cleansing mask: In a small bowl, mix equal parts yogurt or buttermilk and oatmeal. Add one teaspoon of honey and grated apple, if desired. Mix and apply to the face. You may lie down and put warm teabags of chamomile tea on your eyes. Leave on for twenty minutes, and then rinse with warm water. The lactic acid in the yogurt will exfoliate the skin chemically, and the oats will do it physically. A South American variation of this mask adds papaya, which contains a fruit acid that can be an excellent exfoliator and bring beautiful glow to the skin. However, it may be too irritating for damaged or skin sensitized during chemotherapy. If you feel any stinging, wash off immediately with warm water.

Gentle cornmeal exfoliating mask: Mix cornmeal with warm milk and let stand for a few minutes. Use fingertips to work mixture in a circular motion on face and neck. Leave on for ten minutes and rinse thoroughly with warm water. The lactic acid in the milk combined with the corn produces a gentle, natural exfoliation.

Pore-cleansing mask: Combine two tablespoons white clay (kaolin), three tablespoons whipping cream, and one tablespoon rose water to make a paste-like consistency. Spread over clean face, avoiding eye area and lips. Leave on for ten minutes and rinse off with warm water.

Brightening Masks

Skin-brightening mask: Squeeze a squirt of lemon into two tablespoons of honey. Keep in mind that honey will run, so wear an old shirt when applying. Apply to the skin and lie down. After ten minutes, rinse with warm water.

Simple radiance-refreshing mask: Nothing could be easier! Apply pure organic honey to your dry face. Leave for ten minutes, and then rinse off with warm water.

Aloe vera mask (a mask from Anguilla): In a small bowl, mix two tablespoons of honey and two tablespoons of pure aloe plant pulp. (To get the pulp, cut a piece of aloe plant, let the liquid drain a bit, and scoop out the pulp.) Apply to the face and leave on for at least twenty minutes. Rinse with warm water. Because aloe is soothing, raw pulp can be applied directly to skin for minor rashes and acne-like pimples produced by chemo. It can be reapplied often and is safe enough to ingest. It can also be spread all over the body to tighten and moisturize the skin.

Masks for Oily Skin

Yogurt and strawberry mask: Mix natural yogurt and minced fresh strawberries. Apply and leave on for ten to fifteen minutes. The strawberry contains salicylic acid, which is good for unclogging pores.

Orange mask: Slice an orange thinly and apply slices to face. Lie down for ten minutes and rinse with warm water.

Masks for Dry Skin

Orange and egg yolk mask: Mix the juice of half an orange, one egg yolk, one teaspoon sunflower oil, and one teaspoon natural honey. Apply and leave on for ten minutes, and then rinse. This mask is very good for coarse skin.

Baker's yeast mask: Mix three tablespoons baker's yeast with one tablespoon honey. Apply to face and let dry. Rinse with warm water.

Strawberry and egg mask: Combine minced strawberries with one beaten egg. Apply to face and let dry. When dry, apply another layer. Let both layers dry completely, and then rinse with warm water.

Simple yogurt mask: Apply plain yogurt or buttermilk to clean skin. Leave on for ten to twenty minutes, and then rinse with warm water.

Avocado and olive oil: Mix avocado, olive oil, and a few drops of lemon juice. Apply to face and leave on for ten minutes. Rinse with warm water.

Masks for Very Dehydrated Skin

Farmer's cheese mask: Mix two teaspoons farmer's cheese, one teaspoon parsley juice or black tea leaves, and two teaspoons olive oil. Leave on for ten minutes, and then rinse with warm water.

Egg yolk and chamomile mask: Mix one egg yolk, one teaspoon chamomile tea leaves, and a few drops of olive oil. Leave on for ten minutes and wash off with warm, lightly brewed tea.

Chamomile and lavender mask: Mix dried chamomile and lavender leaves, pour hot water over the herbs, and wait until the water is absorbed. Let the mixture stand until the water cools and it is warm but not hot. Apply your favorite cream to your face. Squeeze the excess water from the herbs and spread them over the cream on your face. Lie down and keep the bowl of herbs next to you, putting the mixture over your face periodically. Lay still for about twenty minutes or until the mixture loses its warmth. Remove the mixture and gently wipe the face with a soft cloth to remove remnants.

SPECIFIC SKIN CONCERNS

"Hyaluronic acid (a natural amino acid) may be a solution to acute radioepithelitis [radiation burn], and was used in a double blind clinical study conducted in Switzerland in 1997 on 134 patients undergoing Radiation Therapy. The conclusive findings were 'that a prophylactic use of Hyaluronic Acid is shown to reduce the incidence of high grade radioepithelitis suggesting an interesting role of Hyaluronic Acid as supportive treatments to improve compliance and quality of life in patients undergoing radiation therapy.'" Speak with your dermatologist.
—Kristin Provvidenti, paramedical makeup artist and founder of Stella Bella Pure Active skin care

Radiation Burn

- Radiation burn (radiation dermatitis) is damage to the skin from exposure to radiation, and can be a significant concern for many women of all skin types. It can range from a mild rash, to itchy skin, to open wounds, which can lead to infection. If it is extreme, radiation burn can create long-lasting scarring and hyperpigmentation (darkening). If you develop radiation burn, contact your doctor or dermatologist immediately.

Rosacea

Rosacea is a skin condition that afflicts many adults, and as with any preexisting condition, it can get worse during chemotherapy and/or radiation treatments. Rosacea is tricky to diagnose because it can look like typical acne accompanied by easy flushing, chronic redness on cheeks and nose, or broken blood vessels. Sometimes no pimples form at all. Doctors do not know much about this frustrating disorder, and it is tough to treat. Here are some suggestions:

- Minimize irritating products
- Avoid sun, harsh products, very hot beverages, spicy foods, and red wine.
- Vigorous exercise makes things worse, so take it easier.
- Prescription drugs Metrogel and Finacea can help.
- Oral antibiotics usually targeted for acne may help.

- Over-the-counter soothers include anti-redness products by Skin Effects, La Roche-Posay, and products aimed at sensitive skin.

  - As with most skin conditions during cancer treatment, rosacea is likely to subside a bit after treatment. At that time, you can turn to lasers to minimize broken blood vessels and other hallmarks. See the section "Skin Treatments After Healing."]

Lines and Wrinkles Previously Treated with Botox

Until recently, Botox and other fillers were not recommended during cancer treatment. Now most dermatologists agree that Botox and fillers are OK to use. However, you should avoid them at the height of chemotherapy or when your immune system is very depressed.

Here is why: Botox or fillers themselves are not dangerous, however the delivery method by puncturing the skin with a needle increases the risk of infection. Because chemotherapy (more than radiation) affects cellular activity and may cause wounds to heal more slowly, intentionally wounding the skin with a needle is not a good idea during treatment.

If you do not feel comfortable continuing your Botox and filler treatments, you can still mimic the youth-giving effects in these ways:

- Get a filler treatment before starting chemotherapy/radiation. Fillers in the mid facial area can last six months or even a year.
- During chemotherapy, use topical products that contain ingredients like GABA complex to give a temporary face-lift effect.
- Treat those wrinkle-inducing facial muscles the old-fashioned way by immobilizing them with Breathe Right strips placed over the frown lines between brows during sleep. It really does create a kinesthetic message to the body not to exercise those muscles, according to Dr. Cynthia Bailey. The time-tested antiwrinkle strips Frownies may do the same trick!
- Use plumping moisturizers. Moisturizers containing hyaluronic acid will help keep skin hydrated and plump by increasing the water content of the skin.

- Very gentle exfoliation may also helpful, as this helps stimulate collagen production and gets rid of complexion-dulling dead skin cells, which helps even skin tone and restore luminosity. Dermatologists like ultrasonic skin cleansing brushes like those by Clarisonic. Be sure to sanitize thoroughly after each use, and check with your dermatologist first.
- Get oxygen facials during your treatment. These gentle and relaxing facials, which are finished with pure oxygen spray, leave glowing and refreshed skin. Additionally, they are packed with antioxidants that protect the skin from free radicals. Again, check in with your dermatologist.
- Use vitamin C serum to help rejuvenate the skin.

COSMETIC INGREDIENTS TO AVOID

Today more than ever, thousands of good products address the skin issues brought about by cancer treatments. Nonetheless, the cosmetics industry is still poorly regulated under the Federal Food, Drug and Cosmetic Act (FD & C Act), and cosmetics are the least regulated products. Some formulations have been proven to be toxic and withdrawn from the market *only after* they have been used and consumers have filed complaints. Precaution is the best way to go, particularly when you are undergoing treatment.

The following are some commonly found ingredients in skin care products that you may want to avoid during chemotherapy treatment. Some experts argue that they *are* safe, but they appear time and time again as possible troublemakers. Check in with your doctor.

- *Diethanolamine (DEA)*: DEA is an ethanolamide soap used as a wetting ingredient in lotions and shampoos to give a creamy texture and offer foaming action. It easily penetrates the skin. When your skin is thinned, irritated, or otherwise compromised during treatment, any ingredient that easily gets into the dermis is not good to use. DEA is a known skin irritant but can also convert into nitrosamines, which may be carcinogenic. Avoid DEA and its relatives Oleamide DEA,

Lauramide DEA, and Cocamide DEA, which are commonly used emulsifying or foaming ingredients. Source: *A Consumer's Dictionary of Cosmetic Ingredients* by Ruth Winter, MS (2005).

- *Bronopol*: Bronopol is an antibacterial preservative that can break down into formaldehyde and also may cause carcinogenic nitrosamines. While its use has declined since the 1980s, it may still be used in some high-end cosmetic lines and so-called "natural cosmetics" chains. Be sure to read ingredients.

- *1, 2, 4-dioxane*: Dioxane is a contaminant produced in the manufacturing process and found in a wide variety of shampoos, soaps, and cleansers to produce that satisfying foam we all love. Sometimes it is also found in creams and lotions. Common ingredients that can become contaminated with dioxane are alcohol ethoxylateds, polysorbates, and laureths. A process called "vacuum stripping" can remove dioxane. Dioxane is pretty much nonexistent in organic products certified by the USDA National Organic Program.

- *Silica (quartz)*: Silicon dioxide has been used to improve the feel of foundations, as an anticaking ingredient, and oil absorber. Some debate occurs in the cosmetics community as to whether this type of silica is carcinogenic, but many consider it safe. Still, if only because its proximity in molecular structure to crystalline silica found in asbestos, you may wish to avoid silicon dioxide.

- *Artificial colors*: Water-soluble dyes Blue 1 and Green 3 are carcinogenic, and Green 3 is hardly used any longer. D&C Red 33, FD&C Yellow 5, and FD&C Yellow 6 can harbor cancer-causing impurities as well. Best to steer clear of any product with artificial colors.

- *Sodium laurel, laurel sulfate (SLS)*: This ingredient is everywhere in cleansing products. Obviously, it passes the FDA test because it's so prevalent, but some experts feel it causes skin issues because it strips the skin of oil and thus makes it more prone to irritation and infection.

- *Formaldehyde*: Found in deodorants, nail products, and shampoos, it has been linked with harm to respiratory and immune systems. It is a possible carcinogen.

- *Benzalkonium chloride and benzethonium chloride*: It is found in moisturizers and linked to damage to immune system, and it is a possible carcinogen.

The following ingredients should be avoided at all cost:

- *Talc*: The talcum powder you knew and loved as a child is now known to be a carcinogen linked to ovarian cancer when used in the genital area. Inhaling the powder can pose problems as well, so avoiding its use is best.
- *Saccharin*: Although commonly thought of as a sweetener, it still shows up in some brands of toothpaste. It is linked to bladder cancer.
- *Paraphenylenediamine (PPD)*: PPD can be found in permanent hair dyes, particularly black hair dye. It is also sometimes illegally added to hennas used for temporary tattoos to darken the ink. PPD got a lot of media attention when it was found to be linked to the non-Hodgkin's lymphoma contracted to Jacqueline Kennedy, who had used black hair dye for years. It is considered an allergen that causes dermatitis and secondarily as a carcinogen. But even if it turns out to be nothing more than an allergen, avoid PPD because it's a known skin irritant—and you don't need any more of that.
- *Phthalates*: Phthalates are chemicals produced from oil to create hard plastic and also used as a solvent in cosmetic products such as nail polish (to reduce chipping) and fragrances (to make the scent last longer.) The Environmental Protection Agency (EPA) has determined that phthalates are a "probable human carcinogen." Thankfully, in 2008 Congress passed a law banning the use of phthalates in children's products, and many cosmetics manufacturers have eliminated them from their products. However, phthalates are still around, so look for the following in the products you choose: DBP, DEHP, BzBP, and DMP. Also steer clear of synthetic fragrances.
- *Lead*: Lead occurs rarely in skin care and cosmetics, but can be still found in hair dye for men.

- *Propylene glycol:* This organic substance can be very irritating and has occasionally been linked to dermatitis (rash) and kidney abnormalities.

SPA TREATMENTS DURING HEALING

Spa treatments can be a wonderful boost to body and soul during cancer treatment, but you may need to change the products you use and alter the treatments you usually have at the spa. Safety must be prioritized during the time that your immune system is compromised. The environment of the spa must also support the cancer client. In addition to potentially irritating formulations used by the spa in treatments rooms and overall room scents, infrequent sanitation of rooms and even the detergents used to clean spa linens can affect a patient's immune system that chemotherapy had depressed. Aggressive skin manipulations can also be detrimental.

Anne Willis is a holistic aesthetician and founder of Oncology Skin Therapeutics, which trains aestheticians how to care for skin during cancer treatment. Here are her suggestions to stay safe while relaxing at the spa:

THE BENEFITS OF MASSAGE. *Gentle soft-tissue manipulation of the body with pressure, tension, motion, or vibration targets muscles, tendons, ligaments, skin joints, and connective tissue as well as lymphatic vessels and organs. The benefits associated with body massage include pain relief, reduction of stress and anxiety, and stimulation of the immune and circulatory systems. During chemotherapy and radiation therapy, massage is usually safe and often offers stress release and alleviation of aches and pains while boosting immunities and circulation. Do inform your massage therapist that you are going through cancer treatments. Some salons specialize in chemotherapy massages. Be sure to ask your oncologist if there are any specific reasons you should not get a massage.*

- Be sure you have a good feeling about the facility based on cleanliness, aroma, and the personality of the staff.

- The environment should not be actively simulating: music should be calming and there should be no artificial candles burning or rooms scents.
- Skin needs to be nourished, and this can only be achieved with products that use natural, pure, higher-than-cosmetic-grade ingredients.
- Choose a spa which has experience with cancer patients. Due to skin changes and lowered resistance in the body, patients should be treated by practitioners who have specific training in oncology skin therapies.
- Skin activation should be gentle. Pressure point, lymphatic manipulation and gemstone therapy are the most effective for the oncology client.
- Avoid machines and brushes: they may not be sanitized properly and may be too stimulating to the skin. Also avoid steam: steam machines can be a breeding-ground for bacteria.
- Book your appointments a few days *after* chemotherapy and/or radiation treatment to give you time to monitor your skin's response to the treatment and plan accordingly.

Here are some things to speak about with your aesthetician prior to your treatment:

- Make sure you indicate to the practitioner when you received your last medical treatment. This information can help determine the appropriate spa therapy for you.
- Ask if she has ever worked with clients with compromised immune systems or received specialized training in this area of care.
- Ask her to communicate to you any findings or skin responses she notices.
- Confirm that the treatment will not expose a layer of your skin.
- Ask what products are being used and if they are noncarcinogenic and appropriate for you. It might be best to look for products that are

vegan, green, and organic. (We suggest you call beforehand so you can check out the products' ingredients and avoid wasting valuable appointment time.)

- Ask her to use only disposable sponges and cotton rounds.
- Ask her to clean the product containers. Product containers should be wiped down, especially the neck. Product spills onto these areas during use and can leave excess on the neck, where colonization of bacterium can take place.
- Avoid *more* "chemobrain" drain! End every treatment with written follow-up instructions.

Even if you don't want to try spa treatments, you can use some of the natural, homemade masks we describe at the end of this chapter.

SKIN CARE FOR WOMEN OF COLOR

African-American women suffer similar skin complaints during treatment as do their Caucasian counterparts. The treatments are also similar, with some important additions.

Skin Care Basics

In general, you may wish to follow the CHP routine described above. Here are some other suggestions:

- Use a high-SPF sunscreen *every day* during treatment! Many dermatologists agree that SPF 15 is the minimum; those containing an SPF of 30 might be even better as long as they don't irritate skin.
- Protect lips with a lip balm or serum containing a high SPF.
- Avoid products with irritants such alcohol, dyes, and propylene glycol: irritating the skin can produce an overflow of melanin, increasing the chances for dark spots and pigmentation.

- Avoid products with excessive fragrance.
- If you are prone to blemishes, avoid products containing oil, which can block pores and increase the likelihood of blemishes.
- Avoid alpha hydroxy acids, which can aid in cell turnover and cause uneven pigmentation.
- Keep skin folds dry.

SPECIFIC SKIN ISSUES

Dry Skin

Women of color may experience severely dry skin that takes on a gray or "ashy" look and is more prone to irritation during chemotherapy and radiation. Use extra moisturizing skin treatments.

Radiation Burn

During radiation, women of color may develop more severe radiation-induced dermatitis, a major cause of discoloration. As much as 90 percent of women of color may develop dermatitis, making it a significant concern. Use treatments described above.

DETECTING SKIN CANCER IN WOMEN OF COLOR.

Cancer in darker-skinned people is less understood and can go undetected. Here are two forms of skin cancer that can manifest in dark skin:

Malignant melanoma: This is the most serious form of skin cancer because it can spread so easily to other parts of the body when undetected. For women of color, it is particularly deadly because it often manifests in less exposed areas of the skin such as feet, hands, and nails. Because these spots are less frequently diagnosed, they are mistaken for more common and nonthreatening skin conditions like plantar warts or fungus.

Acral Lentiginous: This is very common form of melanoma in people with dark skin. It is less frequently diagnosed because its symptoms are rather odd. Unlike other skin cancers, which often look like a suspicious spot, acral lentiginous cancer manifests itself as discoloration on the palms or feet or under nails. If you see anything unusual in the coloration of these areas, see your doctor immediately.

As with all cancers, early detection is key to survival, and monthly self-examinations are recommended.

Hyperpigmentation

During chemotherapy, women of color can experience more dark spotting and general skin discoloration, such as vitiligo (loss of pigment), despite the higher concentration of melanin in their skin. These spots and patches can be caused by blemishes, scars, bruises, or cuts that are brought on by the chemotherapy and/or radiation. Says Dr. Debra Jaliman: "Chemotherapy may cause pigmentation that is generalized over the entire body or just limited to certain areas like the palms. It can be caused by a toxic reaction to the melanocytes and they spill their color to the surrounding skin. It occurs two weeks after taking the chemotherapy. It often resolves on its own 3 months after the treatment ends.... It's [very] important to use a broad spectrum sunscreen containing zinc oxide. (SPF 30)."

Hyperpigmentation is notoriously difficult to treat. However, there are variety of ways that can help:

- Wear sunscreen every day.
- Avoid alpha hydroxy acids, which can aid in cell turnover and *cause* uneven pigmentation.
- Avoid products with irritants such alcohol, dyes, and propylene glycol: irritating the skin can produce an overflow of melanin, increasing the chances for dark spots and pigmentation.
- hydroquinone, a skin-lightening compound that works by lessening the concentration of melatonin in the skin, has been shown to help. A dermatologist typically prescribes it, although some over-the-counter creams contain it. The latter are less potent, and effects vary.
- In some cases, retinoids such as Retin-A may be used to help even skin tone.
- Chemical peels may help exfoliate away the discolored skin.
- Creams containing Azelaic acid or kojic acid can be helpful.

Acne

Acne is a very common complaint, and, thankfully, it is also simple to solve. Here are some suggestions from board-certified dermatologist Dr. Tanya Kormeili:

- A variety of lasers and (very light) chemical peels
- Benzoyl peroxide or salicylic acid in light concentrations and which have moisturizers in them. The vehicle (the cream in which the medication is dissolved in) makes a big difference. Recent pharmaceutical advances have helped make many products more tolerable even for dry skins.
- Retinoids
- Topical antibiotics
- Aczone, Finacea (azelaic acid), sodium sulfacetamide, and many combination medicines

Here are some tips:

- Start extra gently with any acne treatment. You can always build up the strength and frequency of the products you use, but it is better to start slowly rather than have to treat a reaction in addition to the acne.
- Try a sonic cleansing machine like those by Clarisonic. They can take most of the bacteria off the skin.
- Keep bed linens and towels scrupulously clean, and keep hair off face while you sleep.

Keloid Scarring

Women of color may be at an increased risk of keloids, which are raised, darkened scars. These scars are difficult (although possible) to treat, and prevention is the best measure:

- Use sunscreen religiously during treatment! We just cannot emphasize this enough.
- Do not pick at blemishes or scars.
- If you do have keloid scars, see a dermatologist as soon as possible. Board-certified dermatologist Dr. Jeanine Downie uses the following treatment: she flattens the scar with a series of cortisone injections, usually once a week, then once every two weeks, then once a month depending on its severity. Laser therapy is then used to build collagen and even out skin tone.

SKIN CARE AND TREATMENTS AFTER HEALING

There is no hard and fast rule about when you can resume your normal skin routines, but it usually about four weeks after chemotherapy or radiation ends. "Check in with your oncologist to find out how long it takes for your body to metabolize and eliminate the chemotherapy drugs before resuming your skin routine," suggests Dr. Fredric Brandt. The same goes for radiation: you do not want to do any treatments on skin that has actually broken down. Wait for your skin to heal thoroughly and then check in with your team. Most dermatologists agree that you can resume the treatments you used before chemotherapy and/or radiation without problems.

Gentle skin care routines you can take will help you emerge from cancer treatment without additional skin changes. However, you may still have "battle scars" that you are unwanted reminders of your healing journey. Many women try new approaches to beauty and wellness after cancer treatment not only to enhance their "new normal," but to remedy any negative cosmetic effects. You may now also want to correct issues that have bothered you even *before* your diagnosis such as fine lines, discoloration, or loss of volume to the face.

Today, there are many restorative medical techniques that address issues like fine lines, creases, skin texture, sagging, or overall rejuvenation. This section talks about restoring your skin after chemotherapy and radiation. It explains today's many dermatologist offerings as well as effective, easy-to-make homemade masks which can be used during treatment, and empowers you to make the best choices for you and your specific issues.

You may find that your treatment has left you with some lasting skin issues, including dullness, or that "aged" look; acne scars and brown spots; more noticeable wrinkles and folds, or new wrinkles; sagging skin; and scars from radiation burn. Here are procedures which can help correct them.

Dullness, or That "Aged" Look

One of the most common side effects of cancer treatment is that skin had lost its former look of health. It may be dry and coarse or now have tiny wrinkles or dullness. It may just look aged from stress. Fortunately, tired-looking skin is one of the easiest issues to treat. Here are some options that are safe, noninvasive, and cost-effective.

Chemical Peels

Chemical peels are very popular: depending on the depth of the peel, they can create smoother, fresher, more radiant skin with little downtime or discomfort. Peels can also slough off minor skin discoloration and blotchiness, help fade acne scars, and erase fine wrinkles. The procedure is also very affordable.

Chemical peels work by mimicking the skin's natural exfoliating process: they hasten the process of skin replenishment by accelerating the production of new skin cells. They remove upper layers of skin and stimulate the deeper layers. Far from being a new science, superficial exfoliation has been used since the time of the Egyptians, when legendary beauty Cleopatra purportedly soaked in sour milk (containing lactic acid) to beautify her skin.

Today, dermatologists use a variety of acids depending on the depth of the peel. These include salicylic acid, Jessner's solution, Resorcinol, trichloroacetic acid, and glycolic or other alpha hydroxy acids (AHA or fruit acid). Sometimes your doctor may pretreat your skin with Retin-A or another retinoic acid for a few days before your peel. This exfoliating agent may help the peel better penetrate the skin.

How Peels Are Performed
- The dermatologist will cleanse and defat (remove oil from) your skin. Acetone or isopropyl alcohol may be used for this purpose because the skin must be completely clear of the makeup or oil that may cause the peel to penetrate unevenly. Then the dermatologist will protect delicate areas, such as lips, with a barrier-like petroleum jelly.
- Next he or she will apply the appropriate acid with a cosmetic sponge or swab. You may feel tingling or slight stinging as the acid is left on your face for the appropriate time period, and a light "frost" will appear. The acid is then washed off with water or neutralized with an alkaline solution such as sodium bicarbonate (baking soda).
- Side effects are few, and healing is relatively simple with peels. You can expect your skin to remain pink the day of and for a few days after the procedure. You may see no visible flaking of the skin, but it will feel firmer and more hydrated. You should absolutely avoid the sun after this or any peel.

An aesthetician in a spa setting does an even gentler version of a superficial peel. Although these peels do not have as dramatic effect as those administered by a dermatologist, they can be a relaxing, pampering treatment that still rejuvenates the skin.

Which Peel Is Right For Me?
The first step is to consult a board-certified dermatologist about which peels are best for your specific skin issues: light, medium-depth, or deep peels.

A Light or Superficial Peel
This in-office procedure typically takes between twenty and forty-five minutes, hence its nickname, "lunchtime peel." It uses mild alpha hydroxy acids that work only on the surface of the skin. Most doctors recommend

a series of these peels to optimize the results: usually four to six treatments spread out over three months or so and correspondingly increasing the strength of the acid used. After this, most dermatologists agree that a treatment every three to four months for maintenance is recommended. Each procedure typically costs between $100 and $250. The procedure is good for overall rejuvenation, very fine wrinkles and lines, and minor dark spots.

Medium-Depth Peel

As the name implies, this is a stronger chemical peel that aims to eliminate old skin cells and therefore produce a more dramatic result. It is often performed with trichloroacetic acid (TCA) and penetrates to the papillary dermis, which lies immediately beneath the epidermis. As with a light peel, after thoroughly cleansing the skin, the acid is applied with a sponge and sometimes massaged in to increase the penetration. This type of peel can cause intense burning, so an analgesia (numbing) cream is often applied before the procedure.

The healing process for this peel is quite a bit longer than for a superficial peel. The skin will brown within a day of the treatment and remain red for a few days after; it will then flake off over the course of the next few to reveal new, brighter skin. You may need to take time off from work and avoid major social engagements while your skin heals. More than one procedure may be recommended, and the cost of this procedure is higher than for a light peel, at around $250 to $750 per session. It is good for deeper wrinkles, brown spots, and acne.

Deep (Phenol) Peel

This is a very aggressive peel recommended only for skin that exhibits *significant* sun damage, wrinkling, deep acne scars, or freckles that need to be removed. It is best reserved for fair skin and is for the face only. It is not an in-office procedure and is performed in a hospital setting under sedation.

A phenol peel penetrates into the dermis, and recovery takes at least ten days, with skin possibly remaining red for as long as two months. It is a serious—and expensive—business that deserves serious consideration and

Fractional Laser Treatment

Fractional lasers are getting a lot of buzz because they do not injure the skin as much as a traditional CO2 lasers, and have less risks and downtime. As the name suggests, the fractional laser treats a fraction of the skin's tissue at a time by creating tiny laser columns that penetrate to the dermis. They address skin texture, fine lines, wrinkles, age or sun spots, acne, and discoloration.

Plasma Laser Treatment

Plasma lasers work by transmitting energy into the dermis without harming the epidermis. They are particularly good for improving the contours of the face and have little downtime.

SPECIALIZED LASERS FOR SPECIALIZED ISSUES.
Lasers work far beyond making skin look better. Here are some examples:
- *unwanted body hair: Alexandrite and Nd: YAG lasers*
- *broken blood vessels: KTP laser*
- *warts: pulsed dye laser*
- *blue veins around eyes: Nd: YAG lasers*

Non-ablative Lasers

Non-ablative laser treatments, unlike the CO2 and Er: YAG lasers, trigger changes within the skin without deliberately damaging or burn the top layer. These gentler treatments have few side effects. As with any treatment, the skin is numbed with an anesthetic cream. During the treatment, your skin may be cooled with liquid nitrogen, so you feel both a cold and hot tingly sensation.

Photofacials

A photofacial is a very gentle laser treatment performed by an aesthetician in a spa environment rather than a dermatologist in an office setting. They are good for brown spots, broken capillaries, boosting collagen, acne, hyperpigmentation, aging skin, and rosacea.

The most common photofacial uses a very narrow spectrum of light to boost collagen and plump up the skin. Other photofacials use intense pulsed light (IPL) lasers. Photofacials are usually quite painless and can be relaxing.

They are typically done in a series of three to four treatments every one to two weeks, with a touch-up every three to four months.

Like laser treatments, photofacials address a number of skin concerns. If you are not ready to commit to the medical procedures outlined above, a photofacial can be a good way to start. Sessions are typically between $250 and $700.

OTHER ANTIAGING TREATMENTS

Thermage

Thermage is a deep-heating radio frequency that, like lasers, stimulates collagen production. It is designed to help sagging skin in many parts of the body. Thermage has grown in popularity and is sometimes used instead of a traditional face-lift or tummy tuck performed by plastic surgeons. It can be a painful procedure, but usually requires just one treatment. It is only good for sagging skin.

Microdermabrasion

Microdermabrasion is a tried-and-true cosmetic treatment that involves spraying the affected skin—which can be the chest, back, arms, or buttocks in addition to the face—with fine aluminum oxide or salt crystals. These particles are then vacuumed up with a gentle suction device. A doctor or someone at a spa can administer the procedure, although those procedures by a doctor may be more aggressive. This mild treatment basically has no downtime.

Microdermabrasion is a much less expensive treatment than lasers and usually costs about $150 to $200 per session. Treatments are recommended two weeks to a month apart for about six months.

It is good for dark spots and acne scars, and can brighten skin and smooth texture.

Vibraderm

Vibraderm is another "sandblasting" technique in which textured, gently vibrating paddles are applied to the skin. These remove layers of damaged skin, revealing healthy, younger-looking skin. This treatment has very little downtime, but the results may be modest. It is a good choice for sensitive skin.

HELP FOR DEEPER WRINKLES: BOTOX AND FILLERS

While chemical peels, lasers, and microdermabrasion can help with smoothing, rejuvenating, and diminishing fine wrinkles, the gold standard to address deeper wrinkles and folds are muscle-weakening injectables such as Botox and fillers. It is good for creases between eyebrows (the so-called "11s"), horizontal lines across the forehead, crow's feet, nasolabial folds (deep smile lines between nose and lips), and creases between lips and chin ("marionette" lines). It can lift eyebrows for a brightening effect.

Botox has become a household name, but its composition and uses bear repeating. Botox is a purified form of botulism toxin and blocks nerve impulses, thereby temporarily freezing facial muscles. It was originally created in the 1970s to treat muscle spasms around the eyes and neck. In 2002 the FDA approved it to treat frown lines.

Botox is injected with a very fine needle into the muscle responsible for the line you wish to soften. This blocks the muscle's ability to move. It does not affect the texture of your skin or how it looks; rather it makes lines less prominent and can erase years from your face.

Botox is generally well-tolerated with few side effects, except for occasional light bruising at the site of the injection. It typically takes a few days for the facial muscles to relax, and depending on how quickly your body metabolizes it, results can last for as long as four months. For some, Botox may have the added benefit of reducing migraines. See your dermatologist for further information. Botox injections typically cost between $400 and $900.

Brand names include Botox, Myobloc, Reloxin (Dysport), and Xeomin.

Fillers

Whereas Botox relaxes facial muscles to smooth existing and deter further creases, fillers do exactly as the name implies: fill in the wrinkles. They are often used in conjunction with Botox. There are both permanent and temporary fillers, which are more popular. Certain types have more targeted applications (mentioned below).

Fillers can give a more natural appearance than surgical procedures by adding volume to the skin. In using dermal fillers, your dermatologist will evaluate your facial appearance and skin tone to determine areas in need of soft tissue augmentation. Strategic points may be marked on your face as guidelines for the injection sites. There are three main kinds: collagen fillers (also called collagen replacement therapy), hyaluronic acid, and those that build collagen in the skin.

A topical anesthetic cream will be applied to your face, and injections are accomplished with a very fine needle. The whole process takes about thirty minutes to an hour. Many different brands of fillers are on the market, and each doctor will have his or her favorite.

Collagen Fillers

Collagen is a protein that occurs in the second layer of skin and makes up most of the skin. It breaks down as a person ages. Collagen replacement therapy restores the natural collagen support layer to your skin. It can be used to plump up lips as well as skin. It is good for smoker's lines around the mouth, marionette lines at the ends of the mouth, worry lines in the forehead, crow's feet at the eyes, deep smile lines, acne scars, cheek depressions or gauntness, dimples, and facial scars.

Harvesting and injecting a patient's own collagen used to be the standard procedure, but now new generations of bovine collagen have grown in popularity. They are safe, well tolerated, and can yield significant results. You will need to take a simple skin test to determine if you're sensitive to the collagen formula. It typically lasts between two and six months. You will receive a topical anesthetic cream as you would with a laser treatment. The injections are accomplished with a very fine needle, and the whole process takes about thirty minutes to an hour. Costs are generally $450 and up.

Brand names include Cosmoplast, Cosmoderm, Zyplast, and Zyderm.

Hyaluronic Fillers

Hyaluronic fillers work on the same principle as collagen fillers. In the skin, hyaluronic acid can bind with water in the tissue, plumping it up. Like collagen, however, the hyaluronic acid in your skin decreases with age. So hyaluronic fillers pump back in the acid, filling in depressions such as acne scars, plumping cheeks or the chin, and filling in lines. The advantage of these kinds of fillers is that they can last twice as long as collagen.

One very popular brand of hyaluronic fillers is Restylane, which is FDA approved. It comes in the form of a gel that is injected into the depleted areas. In addition to being well tolerated, it can last between six and nine months, sometimes even up to eighteen months. Its effects are almost immediate, and it does not shift in the face. It can also be used to plump up lips. At $750 and up, it is not inexpensive, but its staying power can justify the added cost.

Other hyaluronic acid fillers are Perlane, Prevelle Silk, Juvederm Ultra and Ultra Plus, Radiesse (which is also excellent for building volume in thin or aged hands), Artefill, Hylaform, BioForm Radiance, Puragen, and Artecoll (available outside of United States).

Collagen-Building Injectables

Another class of injectable fillers are those that stimulate the body to create collagen around the site of treatment. They are administered like any other injectable. Two of the most popular brands of collagen-building fillers are Sculptra and Radiesse.

Sculptra is made from a type of sugar in the alpha hydroxyl family called Poly-L-lactic acid and is a safe, synthetic, and biocompatible substance that is injected below the surface of the facial skin to provide a gradual yet significant increase in collagen production, improving the appearance of folds and sunken areas.

Sculptra works somewhat differently than other fillers in that it is a powder mixed with water that immediately plumps up when it goes into the body. With each new Sculptra treatment, the skin produces more and more collagen and the results become more permanent. Three or so treatments can last from two to four years. Sculptra is good for building volume over the whole face, even around the eyes, and can also be used for hands. Treatments cost $750 and up.

Radiesse is made from a synthetic version of calcium hydroxylapatite found in teeth and bones. It has been around for a long time for use on damaged vocal cords and to treat urinary incontinence. Unlike Sculptra, Radiesse is a thick white paste containing spheres, which, when injected, stimulates the body to form collagen around them. Although it is recommended for deep lines around the mouth, it is not recommended for lips. Radiesse costs about the same as other fillers, can last about a year.

Permanent Fillers

Some permanent fillers are available, such as fat injections (LipoStructure, TDL [Transconjunctival Deep Lipotransfer]), liquid inject-able silicone, and Artefill/Artecoll Dermal Filler. These procedures deserve serious consideration and consultation with an experienced dermatologist, as they are lifetime commitment—and a very costly one at that. For some women, however, they are ideal. Speak to your doctor.

COST CONSIDERATIONS FOR MEDICAL COSMETIC PROCEDURES

Many women put off voluntary dermatological and spa treatments because of the cost. However, here are some things to consider:

- Despite its immediate expense, a proven medical treatment for your skin issue may save you money in the long run. Not only it might cost less than you think, it might replace the expensive products you cur-rently use that are not cost-effective in comparison.
- Many cosmetic dermatologists will work out an appropriate payment plan for their patients. Do not be afraid or embarrassed to ask about alternative payment arrangements when you discuss your treatment!
- Emotions count. Effectively resolving your skin issues will have a real emotional benefit. Start banking money for your treatment, so if you do have trouble justifying it as a one-time expense, you will feel you earned it.
- Time matters. You might not get the results you want with an over-the-counter product no matter how good it is, and you might invest time in waiting for a result that will not be satisfactory. Sometimes solving an issue quickly will have more of a benefit than waiting it out.

LOW-TECH OPTIONS

If you do not wish to do a skin treatment and prefer something at home, here are suggestions from dermatologists.

Sallow/aged skin

- A glycolic acid antiaging skin care regimen based on your skin type
- At-home microdermabrasion such as DermaNew Microdermabrasion Total Body Experience

Age spots

- Prescription Solagé cream
- DERMADoctor Immaculate Correction

Broken capillaries

- Prescription MetroGel or Finacea cream

Lines and creases

- Topical line relaxers (TLRs) that give a Botox-like effect
- DERMAdoctor Immobile Lines
- Dr. Brant Crease Release

Loss of volume, wrinkles, and depressions

- DERMAdoctor Faux Fillment
- Or, for at-home, natural remedies you can try some of our homemade masks, below.

Frequently Asked Questions about Skin Care

Should I really be worried about my skin at this time?

Even if you think worrying about your skin during a time of crisis is vain, paying attention to symptoms is very important to your medical care. Dr. Mario Lacouture, onco-dermatologist: "If significant skin reactions are not managed quickly, dose interruptions, reductions, or discontinuation of chemotherapy and/or radiation can occur, thus impacting clinical outcomes for the patient...Chronic skin inflammation undermines all levels of healing."

Could all the stress of cancer treatment itself have aged my skin?
Yes. This may, in fact, have nothing to do with the chemotherapy drugs themselves. Recent studies have shown that stress and tension alone can affect cells located beneath the skin surface, resulting in a decrease in elasticity and deeper facial lines.

Dr. George Murphy, professor of dermatology and pathology at the University of Pennsylvania, states: "After all, if stress can bring forth unwanted changes such as premature graying of hair, wouldn't it promote wrinkles?" Another study in 2004 showed a link between constant worry and accelerated skin aging. Stress actually slows down the cell renewal process. It also does more dangerous things such as weakening the immune system, impacting our heart and disrupting much-needed sleep.

A few key steps can help lessen your body's response to stress:

- Exercise: while most experts agree that thirty minutes of aerobic activity a day is best, even a simple walk a day can do you good.
- Revamp eating habits with the help of a nutritionist.
- Stay hydrated: in addition to helping with the effects of stress, it plumps up the skin.
- Think about pampering yourself with a rejuvenating treatment that will make you feel better about the way you look. Looking in the mirror and feeling great will go a long way to boosting your self-esteem and banishing some stress!

With skin care products, is natural always better?
In general, doctors agree that natural ingredients are less irritating to the skin and can be safer as well. However, there are always exceptions. Dr. Noëlle Sherber: "Poison ivy is natural, so natural doesn't always mean nonirritating! [For example]...one of the biggest misconceptions that patients

have when going through chemotherapy or radiation is that aloe vera gel is a good skin soother. It can actually be a…cause of contact dermatitis, particularly when used on sensitive skin. Some patients who get hot flashes with treatment like to use cooling gel on their skin, but a hypoallergenic kept in the refrigerator would be a better choice than aloe."

Dr. Shannon Trotter adds: "Natural does not always mean safe or good. It may sound better or more attractive, but a lot of natural ingredients can be irritating to the skin or cause an allergic reaction. It's better to look for a treatment that meets the needs of the patient and not simply choose it based on having natural ingredients."

Our best advice? Use your judgment, honor your personal philosophy, and check in with your oncology team.

Can supplements help?
Dr. Elena Klimenko: "Good nutritional support during the chemo and radiation will provide the body with all necessary substances to keep skin healthy and heal the inflammation faster. The most important are adequate amount of proteins, preferable in predigested, easily utilized form like amino acids, specially glutamine; fish oil and omega-3, -6, and -9; and powerful antioxidants: glutathione, selenium, vitamin C, and the probiotic Aristophanes."

Try topical antioxidants too. Dr. Fredric Brandt suggests: "To boost skin glow while undergoing treatments, we recommend high doses of topical antioxidants (i.e., green tea, grape seed, etc.). These can reduce radical damage that may be occurring."

My chemo cocktail has caused permanent dark spots and broken blood vessels. What treatment can help?
Dr. Jeanine Downie: "The Excel V laser is excellent for these. It rejuvenates the skin and is safe and effective for all skin types."

Moisturizing? Hydrating? What's the difference?
While people tend to use the terms interchangeably, moisturizing and hydrating formulations are different and each addresses a different skin

issue. Moisturizers (also called emollients) are designed to soften the top layers of skin and increase its water content by preventing loss of water. They are occlusive, which means they create a barrier between the skin and environment to prevent loss of moisture. Moisturizers tend to be oil-based, contain humectants (ingredients that attract and hold in moisture), and lubricants (which reduce friction and therefore irritation).

Hydrators, on the other hand, do not contain oil and are designed for skin that already has enough oil but still needs moisture content. An example of this is skin that is internally oily, but superficially dry due to stripping by harsh cleansing agents, windburn, etc. Hydrators are water-based and restore and maintain the skin's water balance, therefore making them better choices for women with oily or acne prone skin.

What are the protocols for bathing now that my skin is drier?
Dr. Shannon Trotter: "Patients should follow a skin-care routine that includes taking daily lukewarm showers or baths limited to fifteen minutes. Soap should be used sparingly and only in areas that tend to perspire or become dirty, such as the body fold areas."

I'm getting chemo, but people are telling me I look healthy and sun-kissed!
Pigmentation—either all over or in areas—can be a side effect of chemotherapy and is commonly referred to as "chemo tan." It tends to appear two to three weeks after the start of treatment. Certain chemotherapy drugs are more likely to produce this temporary effect (see our appendix). While it is still uncertain why these particular drugs make you look tan, it is thought that they may increase melanin production by stimulating melanocytes.

Unfortunately, there appears to be no treatment for temporary hyperpigmentation except the use of hydroquinone in some cases. But the good news is that hyperpigmentation and "chemo tan" usually disappear as new skin cells replace the dead cells around ten to twelve weeks after the conclusion of treatment. Use of sunscreen is *vital* during chemotherapy to minimize hyperpigmentation.

What are some sunscreens suggested by a dermatologist?
Dr. Jeanine Downie: "The main source of skin damage and scarring is the sun: sun protection is an absolute must *regardless of ethnicity!* Use sunscreen with an SPF of at least 30 every day, rain or shine. Some good ones include SkinMedica Daily Physical Defense, Diorsnow UV Shield White Reveal Moisturizing UV Protection SPF 50, and Neutrogena Ultra Sheer Dry-Touch Sunscreen, SPF 55."

I'm having hot flashes, and cooling creams do not seem to work. Can medication help?
More and more we are learning how drugs can multitask: Botox was developed for chronic pain but is now used to treat wrinkles; anti seizure medications such as lamotrigine (Lamictal) are very effective in treating bipolar disorder; and guanfacine (Tenex), a medication to treat high blood pressure, is successfully used to treat ADHD. So it should come as no surprise that an anti-anxiety, antidepressant can treat menopausal symptoms! According to Dr. Mario Lacouture, venlafaxine (Effexor) has been helpful in treating hot flashes and night sweats you may experience during chemotherapy. Speak to your doctor.

I detect a chemical scent on my body from chemo: what should I do?
First, switch to a nonmetallic deodorant, particularly if you are undergoing radiation in the breast area. Start carrying gentle baby wipes with you to freshen your skin. Be sure to use ones that are natural and free of preservatives and fragrance. Don't be alarmed if your urine takes on a chemical scent too. Baby wipes can help with this as well.

I have bad acne scars from chemotherapy and have heard of a new technique using a roller. What is this?
The Microneedle Therapy System is a new treatment to help skin needing resurfacing, and it can be very effective for acne scars. It is literally a roller loaded with tiny needles that is moved over the skin—much like you would move a lint roller over clothing. When the device is rolled, it forms

microchannels in the skin. These tiny wounds stimulate the body to heal them and form new skin.

The manufacturer's claim is that Microneedling is more effective than ablative lasers or microdermabrasion for smoothing wrinkles, removing acne scars, and reducing the appearance of stretch marks. They also claim it is virtually free of side effects except for slight redness to the skin for a few hours after treatment. Although the rollers are available online, speak with your dermatologist before purchase.

What chemotherapy drugs are likely to cause neuropathy?
Some chemotherapy drugs that may cause chemotherapy-induced peripheral neuropathy (CIPN) are vincristine, cisplatin, paclitaxel, and the podophyllotoxins (etoposide and teniposide), thalidomide, and interferon. Although there have been many medical studies about treatment for this painful condition, few have been found: "Agents with the strongest supporting evidence for efficacy in the treatment of CIPN include topical pain relievers, such as baclofen/amitriptyline/ketamine gel, and serotonin and norepinephrine reuptake inhibitors, such as venlafaxine and duloxetine" ("Chemotherapy-Induced Peripheral Neuropathy: Prevention and Treatment." CL Loprinzi, DR Pachman, DL Barton, and JC Watson. *Clinical Pharmacology & Therapeutics*. 2011 September, 90(3): 377–387). See your doctor immediately. He or she may prescribe a full physical and neurological examination to determine if the neuropathy is a result of an underlying cause such as diabetes.

The acne that started with my chemotherapy treatment refuses to go away! I don't want to have lasers, and topical medications are not helping much. Is there anything else?
One new device is called the Isolaz Acne Light System which is very effective for blackheads, whiteheads, and sometimes even cystic acne. Think of it like a safe and gentle vacuum cleaner for your skin. The treatment starts with a careful steaming of the face to open pores, and then uses a gentle suction

device to remove impurities and unclog pores. It is finished with another steam. Four to five treatments may be suggested. There is no downtime, and the effects can be impressive.

Can someone besides my dermatologist please describe what a photofacial is like? Lana Koifman, founder of Surviving Beautifully: "Absolutely! I am a big fan of photofacials, which are done at a spa using the Sciton BBL laser. It's easy and quick. First, I put on the numbing cream, which feels cool and grainy. In twenty minutes, my skin feels numb. I barely feel anything when the photofacial is performed. At worst, I feel a 'rubber band snap' sensation. The whole thing takes about thirty-five to forty minutes.

"After the numbing cream wears off, my skin feels as if I have a mild sunburn, kind of hot and tingly. This feeling can last anywhere from an hour to several hours depending on the intensity of the procedure. However, I can easily go back to work or go out at night. But I would not plan this procedure very close to a major event, as over the next few days, the spots on my face (age spots and freckles) get very dark. This can be barely noticeable to quite noticeable. In another few days, the spots naturally slough off. Toward the end of the week, my skin is clear. This is a wonderful procedure to get after cancer treatments, as the chemo enhanced my freckles. This treatment truly makes them go away!"

Some people get sensitive to fragrances during chemo, but I'm not. I know that fragrance-free products are recommended, but do I really need to give up my favorite scents? Dr. Shannon Trotter: "I don't ignore how hard it is for some patients to trade in their lotion for a bland product. Their lives have already changed dramatically, and something like their vanilla-scented lotion may be one of the few normal things they have left. I simply tell my patients that these [moisturizing] products are not sufficient to maintain skin hydration and they also carry a risk of irritation. However, I encourage my patients to purchase the body splash or perfume instead and apply sparingly. This is an important part to help them maintain their identity and femininity. I know how important a woman's perfume can be, and I try not to take that away."

I have a mild rash and would prefer to use something low-tech. Any suggestions?
Long ago humankind discovered that leaving grapes to ferment produced wine, but leaving wine out to sour creates vinegar. White vinegar has been used for thousands of years as a cleansing agent. It also reduces bacteria and is proven to help with localized itching from radiation dermatitis or all-over itch. Pour two cups of white vinegar into a lukewarm—not hot!—bath and soak for a bit. Or make a compress of diluted vinegar and apply to the affected area. Always check in with your dermatologist first.

What is compounding, in terms of skin treatment?
Compounding simply means creating a unique pharmaceutical product depending on the patient's needs. During cancer treatment, doctors often compound medications for skin care: "For example, if a patient experiences significant itch associated with their skin, we can compound products with menthol. Compounding offers a unique opportunity to become creative and really cater to your patient," says Dr. Shannon Trotter.

I have heard a lot about the benefits of white mud. What is it?
Several Eastern European breast cancer survivors we interviewed talked about this mysterious substance that is excellent at cleansing the skin and drawing out toxins during chemotherapy and hormone therapy. It turns out that "white mud" is also known as French White Powder Clay (kaolin). It is an old-world cosmetic ingredient known for its ability to absorb and clear the skin of excess oil and waste. You can buy it in bulk on the Internet. Using it is easy: simply mix with water to make a paste, smooth on face (or body), let dry, and gently remove with tepid water.

I anticipate that I'm going to look pale and tired while undergoing treatment. Is it safe to use a self-tanner?
Dr. Maria Theodoulou: "If these products are used appropriately—not on the whole body, not every day—then it can be nice to have a tan on those exposed parts of the body when you're undergoing chemotherapy to avoid the chemo pallor. It can be safe if used sparingly. There are times when

Ever notice when you use often lip balm containing petrolatum that your lips feel chapped and dry without it? That's because petrolatum interferes with the body's own moisturizing process and ironically creates the very symptoms it is supposed to alleviate.

Using products containing ceramides, the natural lipid of the skin, may be better. Says Dr. Tanya Kormeili: "Ceramides reduce inflammation and help restore the skin epidermis. There are [prescription] moisturizers: Hylatopic Plus and EpiCeram. There are also over-the-counter ceramide products: CeraVe is the most popular. Eucerin and Cetaphil are also light but effective moisturizers containing ceramides."

My hands and feet are numb, and then they itch and burn. What is going on?
You may have hand-foot syndrome. This condition is caused by small amounts of chemotherapy drug that leak out of very small blood vessels in the palms of the hands and soles of the feet. Your palms and feet may be red, tender, peeling, and numb.

If you suspect you have hand-foot syndrome, see your doctor, who may prescribe vitamin B6 or a prescription cream to help. Also some new research indicates that an antidepressant may help. The good news is that hand-foot syndrome tends to disappear a few weeks after the treatment.

Here are some suggestions to minimize the symptoms:

- After you start chemotherapy treatment, avoid long exposure of hands and feet to hot water. Instead, take short showers in tepid water.
- Try to avoid wearing unlined gloves for washing dishes, as the rubber will hold heat against your palms.
- Avoid increased pressure on the soles of the feet, like jogging, aerobics, power walking, jumping, or long days of walking.
- Avoid using garden tools, household tools such as screwdrivers, and other tasks where you are squeezing your hand on a hard surface.
- Avoid using knives to chop food, which may also cause pressure and friction on your palms.

To alleviate symptoms of hand-hoot syndrome, consider the following:

- Place the palms or bottoms of your feet on an ice pack or a bag of frozen peas. Alternate on and off for fifteen to twenty minutes at a time.
- For feet, gel soles like those by Dr. Scholl's may be helpful.
- Try Elasto-Gel Hot/Cold Therapy Wraps and Carrington Medical Gel Packs.
- Use an emollient cream to help with dryness and avoid further irritation.

Is there anything I can do to help my eyes appear less puffy in the morning?
Yes. Train yourself to sleep on your back to reduce puffiness. A form-fitting or buckwheat-filled pillow may be helpful. Another trick is to use ice cubes in the morning to "wake up" the eyes. Makeup artist Cindy Barbakov recommends massaging the eye area with ice cubes for two minutes, which can freshen up the eye area and even make the whites look brighter.

What are parabens, and are they carcinogenic?
In scientific terms, a paraben is a quaternary ammonium compound or ethyl or isopropyl alcohol used as a preservative. It can penetrate the skin and bind to estrogen receptors, thus raising estrogen levels. According to *A Consumer's Dictionary of Cosmetic Ingredients* by Ruth Winter, parabens are endocrine disrupters (EDs) that are thought to act like the female hormone estrogen, which, in high quantities, can cause some women to develop breast cancer. The most commonly used forms are methyl-, propyl-, and parahydroxybenzoate. Check out your medicine cabinet—these guys are everywhere! In fact, you can find them in a whopping 70 to 90 percent of all shampoos, makeup, lotions, and deodorants.

Perhaps natural preservatives are safe and we should simply turn to our local organic and health food store. But wait: tons of plant endocrine disrupters are out there as well. Called phytoestrogens, these occur in herbs such as St. John's Wort, hops, dong quai, sage, and red clover and in pumpkin, using lip balms made from only active moisturizing ingredients, and my favorite lip hydrating ingredient is shea butter."

Cancer treatments didn't affect my face, but I now have dark spots and wrinkling on my body. Help!
Try a chemical peel. Unlike other cosmetic procedures like fillers and Botox, chemical peels can be used on many parts of the body. They can help with light wrinkling or loss of radiance, and they are ideal for spot treatments for discoloration at radiation sites, acne scars, sun spots, or warts. Speak with your dermatologist.

Is there a way to protect my lips from the sun besides protective lip balm?
Dr. Jeanine Downie: "Yes. In a pinch, you can just rub regular sunscreen for the face into lips and seal in with a coat of Vaseline or Aquaphor."

What can I do to boost glow?
Dr. Fredric Brandt recommends a very light peel in certain cases to boost skin's glow. Some controversy exists because peels can cause the inflammation, which, ironically, is what helps the skin rejuvenate. Ask your doctor.

Everyone says to stop using Retin-A during chemotherapy, but my skin can handle it and it's the only thing that helps my acne.
Dr. Noëlle Sherber: "If your skin is accustomed to prescription-strength tretinoin (Retin-A, Atralin, ReFissa), then switching to a milder over-the-counter retinol can be a good choice. Products containing peptides such as Matrixyl and Dermaxyl build collagen in the same way tretinoin does. While not as strong as tretinoin, they have studies to support their efficacy and don't have the potential to cause irritation in the way that prescription retinoids can."

How do dermatologists treat rashes from radiation?
Dr. Tanya Kormeili: "Radiation causes inflammation, and it is these inflammatory cells that damage the pigment cells and cause discoloration. We give

our patients deep moisturizers and cortisone and anti-inflammatory products to minimize inflammation. If you do have scarring, see your dermatologist as soon as possible."

Chemotherapy has brought on acne, but I'm too sensitive for acids like glycolic acid. What can I look for in terms of ingredients that won't irritate?
Paramedical makeup artist and founder of Stella Bella skin care, Kristin Provvidenti: "A common denominator in many skin conditions is keratinization—a buildup of protein on the skin and within the pores. This protein production can be accelerated when undergoing treatment. As cells lose moisture and are pushed up toward the surface of the skin, they stick to the walls of the pores by way of the sticky protein. This is the purpose of using alpha and beta hydroxy acids like glycolic acid. Because glycolic acid has the smallest molecular structure with one atom molecule as opposed to two or three of salicylic or lactic, it penetrates deeper and may cause irritation. Salicylic, having a larger molecular structure, is often a better choice for those struggling with oily skin but can be irritating to compromised skin as well.

Aspen bark is a derivative of salicylic acid. It is markedly weaker and therefore a more gentle option. Aspen bark has been used for centuries by Native American Indians as an analgesic as well as to treat burns, eczema, and other skin conditions. Stella Bella, for example, uses pure aspen bark in our oily skin formulations."

What can I do about scars from radiation treatment?
Scars from radiation and sometimes chemotherapy can be some of the longest-lasting, and most distressing, reminders of your fight with cancer. Dermatologist Dr. Jeanine Downie has these suggestions:

- Deal with any scarring immediately. It sounds counterintuitive, and most people assume a scar should heal completely before any cosmetic treatment, but the newer and fresher the scar, the easier it is to manipulate and fix. Plus you may end up needing to have more treatments—and therefore spend more money—if you wait.

- For scars from radiation burn, I use the Fraxel Re: pair laser in particular.
- A prescription cream like Biafine can really help with radiation scarring if you don't want to use lasers, and insurance usually covers it. Make sure whatever treatment you choose, to use a gentle cleanser on the area. Good drugstore brands include Dove, Cetaphil, and Aveeno.

I know lasers can help with dark scars, but what about the light scars (and loss of pigment) I have?

Yes. The XTRAC laser, originally developed to treat psoriasis, can help repigment the skin of patients with vitiligo, or pigment loss, and also white stretch marks. It delivers monochromatic UVB right to the affected area, thereby restoring pigmentation without damaging the surrounding healthy skin area (as you would with UVB gotten through sun exposure).

I have acne from my chemotherapy cocktail—shouldn't I be using a stronger cleanser?

Dr. Cynthia Bailey: "When women going through chemo begin to get oily skin accompanied by acne, it is common to think you need to use products that lather heavily and leave the skin feeling 'squeaky' clean. Unfortunately, by doing so, often the delicate acid mantle is washed away, leaving skin even more vulnerable. The body produces this acid mantle to protect the skin, keep moisture in, and eliminate acne-born bacteria that thrive in an alkaline environment. If it lathers heavily, it most likely is more alkaline than acidic."

Kristin Provvidenti adds: "One of the most important things I feel is to be sure that you use products that are pH correct. Some of the most recommended acne soaps have a pH factor of 11 or more, which is right in line with Comet cleanser! The body then goes into 'protection mode' by trying to reestablish this acid mantle and the skin, while drier under the top layers of the epidermis, becomes even more oily at the surface."

I heard the biofeedback machine can help with skin problems. Really?
Maybe! Cancer survivor Lena A. is from Russia and, by accident, discovered an unusual tool that really helped her skin during cancer treatment. Called Scenar in the United States, it is a biofeedback pain management device created by OKB RITM Russia, a medical innovator that started out creating technologies for space. It emits a harmless electrical impulse that stimulates the body's own pharmacy via the skin, helping to relieve and manage pain, and is also now used in the Russian beauty market. Lena found it made her face glow, even during the ravages of chemotherapy. It is expensive at around $700, but could be the thing if pain management is also part of your regimen. The company also makes therapeutic blankets. For more information, visit www.scenar-usa.com.

I want to use a really low-tech product to moisturize my skin. What can I make at home?
Makeup artist Dee Dee Jones: "Turn coconut oil into a skin treatment by mixing a few drops of essential oils with coconut oil and blend for several minutes in a food processor. This makes a rich body balm: it really is divine and feels like an expensive luxury cream!" Works great on lips too.

I know what I'm supposed to avoid in skin-care products, but what are some natural ingredients to look for?
Jennifer Young, biochemist and founder of Defiant Beauty skin care for cancer patients: "Cancer patients don't need me to tell them that they have very sensitive skin. Their skin now reacts to all kinds of products that, pretreatment, had been firm favorites. When deciding on a product to use through and post-treatment, simple products with few ingredients are the key. Ingredients like apricot kernel oil and peach kernel oil are traditionally used for sensitive skin, but as anyone can react to anything, there is no guarantee that one won't react. Patch tests are vital when deciding upon a product, natural or otherwise. Good manufacturers will facilitate this; some even allow patch testing of the ingredients. This allows you to identify ingredients that you are sensitive to, thus enabling you to avoid them in all products."

What are the benefits of the natural oils cropping up everywhere?
Jennifer Young: "The benefits of natural oils are many. Oils are much more concentrated than creams and lotions, which are mostly water. As soon as water is removed from a product, cosmetic biochemists like myself are able to discard many other 'chemical' ingredients. Even natural creams and lotions contain preservatives, emulsifiers, pH adjustors, conditioners, etc. They are required, because creams and lotions contain both oil and water, which don't mix naturally and need a helping hand. These 'helping hands' are additional ingredients and increase the likelihood of a sensitive-skinned person reacting to the beauty product. For example, cancer patients often suffer irritated skin as a result of their treatment. Our Itchy Skin Oil (named by the patients and survivors who asked me to create the range) contains oils such as calendula and St. John's Wort. They are known for their healing and soothing properties, and clinical oncology trials have shown calendula oil to be an effective treatment for radiation damaged skin."

I'm concerned about all the synthetic ingredients in sun block. Can you explain more and give some safe suggestions?
Kristin Provvidenti: "The problem with using chemical sun protections often found in moisturizers or other creams is that the active ingredients, usually in the benzone or cinnamate family, are actually derived from petroleum. This can cause acne in some people and can also act as an irritant. Avobenzone, oxybenzone, and many other chemical sunscreen ingredients work by absorbing the solar rays and dispersing them as heat on the skin's surface. This can exacerbate inflammation and redness, increasing capillary dilation. Because of the way sunscreens work on the skin, they metabolize quickly and need to be 'slathered' on in larger amounts than most women are comfortable with. They also need to be reapplied often to be effective.

"Using a sunscreen with zinc oxide and/or titanium dioxide is a better alternative. However, most creams containing these ingredients leave the skin looking chalky. More and more companies have remedied this look by using micronized zinc or titanium dioxide.... We use high micron zinc oxide and titanium dioxide in our formulations, offering broad spectrum protection, and unlike most mineral powders available, we do not incorporate the common filler bismuth oxychloride in our formulas, which is a heavy metal derived from copper and smelt refining, similar to arsenic in molecular structure and a known irritant and skin sensitizer.

"For women who are going to be in the sun for extended periods of time, like a trip to the beach, I recommend Badger Brand Sunscreens, which are natural, organic, and don't incorporate micronized titanium or zinc in their products."

Can you give me a simple but delicious recipe to support skin health?
Lisa Grey, creator of Pink Kitchen, a website devoted to nutritional support during cancer treatment, suggests you also treat your skin from within: "To make our bodies an unfriendly environment for cancer to grow, we need to practice good nutrition. For example, age spots ('sun spots') are often an outward sign that we are storing toxins on the inside. However, antioxidants and certain vitamins and minerals, such as vitamin C and selenium, may help to fade existing age spots and prevent future age spots. The best source of antioxidants, vitamins, and minerals is not from a bottle, but from eating fresh vegetables and fruits several times per day. Here's a recipe to start:

Quinoa with Spinach & Brazil Nuts
  Yield: 4 servings

  ½ tsp. allspice
  1 c. Brazil nuts
  1 small bag of spinach leaves
  3 cloves garlic, minced
  ¼ c. olive oil
  sea salt to taste

Prepare 4 servings of quinoa according to package directions, adding allspice to the water. Crush Brazil nuts so that you have some large pieces, but mostly small pieces. Sauté garlic and Brazil nuts in olive oil over low heat. Add spinach, stirring until just wilted.

"The skin at my radiation site was very tender. What kept me comfortable was wearing the softest men's T-shirt I could find. I cut the sleeves off and wore it against my skin with my bra tight over it. It was soft and didn't move."
—VJ Sleight

"My eyes felt dry and stingy after chemo. I would lie down in the evening with warm tea bags on my eyes. And whenever I felt especially tired and my joints hurt, I would put a white mud [kaolin] mask over my whole body, including my face. I would wash it off after about twenty minutes and then soak in a warm tub." —Lana Koifman

"Using an oil or serum on the skin, as well as a moisturizer, will help the skin absorb the product more easily, therefore being more effective, and if the side effects of chemo are dreary eyes and loss of smell, facial massage using a suitable facial oil (ideally with rose oil/rosehip, as it's super for the skin) can also help with the this." —Cindy Woodward, skin-care therapist at the Beauty Retreat Organic Day Spa, Sheffield, England, and caregiver for a cancer patient

"Drink lots of water; it is good for you and your skin." —Tiffany Reuter

"To treat hand-foot syndrome and keep my fingernails and toenails, I iced my hands during my chemo infusions. For the next two days I put my hands and feet into ice baths for twenty minutes three times a day." —Heidi Bright, M. Div., www.heidibright.com

"I was very fortunate that my skin remained healthy during treatment... [T]he only bummer was I picked a small pimple while undergoing chemo, and it took forever to heal! I now have permanent scar in that spot. I avoided 'picking' after that!" —Krista Colvin, www.puttingonmybiggirlpanties.com

"Oxygen therapy facials are amazing for the skin. Medical consent should be sought just to be on the safe side, but as it's pure oxygen and product-infusion involved, there should not be any reason why it would not be given." —Cindy Woodward

"I used a beeswax-based hand and foot bar from a local beekeeper to reduce the roughness and chapping on my hands and feet." —Heidi Bright

"When I was diagnosed, my aesthetician told me she was now in charge of my skin. I had facials every three weeks, and it made a *huge* difference with my personal mental health as well as my skin care. She told me she understands that the cells responded well to peptides.

"She also worked on my 'port,' and to this day, it is hard to tell what that blemish on my chest was; usually it is a telltale sign of cancer world." — Cindy Giles, Cancer Coach

"Cancer treatment can wreak havoc on your complexion…acne, blackheads, clogged pores, and the like. Try Aztec Secret Indian Healing Clay. This 100 percent calcium bentonite clay has been dubbed the 'world's most powerful facial.' Almost every mineral found on Earth is present in this volcanic ash. It's 100 percent natural and boasts over fifty skin-healing and nourishing minerals that literally pull all the yucky stuff out of your pores.

"Simply mix equal parts of the powder with warm water or raw apple cider vinegar in a glass or plastic bowl. (Do not use metal, as this interacts with the clay.) I mix mine in a plastic zip baggie so I can refrigerate it and use any leftover mixture at a later time. Apply the mud to your face and other areas of your body and let it sit for ten to twenty minutes before washing off with warm water. The absolute max to leave it on is forty-five minutes. You can use it once or twice a week, and up to three times a week for problematic skin. You will feel tightening as the mask hardens, and your skin may be red afterward; this is completely normal, so don't be alarmed. You can also put a few scoops in your bathwater to help detoxify the skin. Aztec Secret Indian Healing Clay is available online and in health food stores for under $10. It's amazing!" —April Dawn Ricchuito, www.verbal-vandalism.com

"I used coconut oil on my entire body and paid special attention to scars because if my skin was dry, the scars would widen. It's important to massage and keep the scares from becoming too dry. I actually still use the coconut oil for my entire body." —Gaye Moore Lewis

"If you have dry eyes, try Genteal eye gel. It's thicker than drops and distributes better in your eyes. Also, switch to glasses instead of contacts before starting chemo." —Dawn A. Gum

"For laundry detergent, I use Ava Anderson nontoxic." —Wendy Kuhn, cancer survivor and holistic health coach, www.breakthroughconsultingllc.com

"I put vitamin E on my eight-inch scar after my liver surgery. It helped to reduce the redness and heal the skin." —Ivelisse Page

"Dermatology, allergy, and asthma clinicians use a method for treating terrible eczema and psoriasis in children and adults called 'soak and seal,' which I adopted during my radiation treatments to help severe redness and blistering. My skin blistered after the second week, and I had six weeks left to go. The radiation nurse honestly did not think I would be able to finish without taking a week off. But I started soak and seal and also a green tea mask and was able to get it under control in less than a week. Consequently I finished thirty-two treatments on schedule!

Soak and Seal
- Fill your tub with about one to two feet of water or more (not too hot).
- Sit in the tub with a very wet washcloth or hand towel (depending on the size of the affected area) and apply it right on the burned skin. Use a small cup and keep the washcloth wet by pouring water on it frequently over a twenty-minute period. Don't get out of the tub until the skin on your fingers is wrinkled.
- When you get out, lightly pat your affected skin dry and then apply a thick layer of moisturizer. Really slather it on. I use Vanicream and

Vaniply, which can be purchased at the pharmacy, or you can use any other high-quality skin cream.

Green Tea Mask

This is something else that really helped my blistered and burned skin. You need to use matcha green tea, which is a finely powdered tea available at natural food stores.

- Take a small dish and mix about two to three tablespoons of the green tea with one tablespoon of honey mixed with a little water until you get a think, clay-like consistency.
- Apply the green tea mask on your burned skin and let it soak in for about fifteen minutes, and then rinse it off.
- I often did this first in the tub, and then did Soak and Seal because it is a little messy.

"These two techniques helped me get through radiation." —Jori Walker

NAIL CARE DURING CANCER TREATMENT

Like your skin, your nails can also experience changes during chemotherapy. However, like many other side effects of chemotherapy, nails will very likely grow out normally after treatment. Certainly some chemotherapy cocktails can cause more nail issues than can others, so speak with your oncology team if you notice significant side effects such as unusual bleeding, discharge, or pain.

You might experience the following:

- Changes in nail color, like darkening and discoloration (pigmentation) (Adriamycin and Cytoxin especially can cause this)
- Nails split or become brittle and chip easily
- Nails become softer or shed (onycholysis)
- Nails lift off the nail bed. While this is more uncommon, it requires you to be extra careful. For one thing, the nail may fall off entirely,

leaving the nail bed exposed and tender. A partially lifted nail can harbor bacteria and lead to infection because it's no longer securely attached to the nail bed.

- Nails have a horizontal line: this is relative to your chemotherapy schedule and will grow out as your treatments stop. Sometimes you may experience deep horizontal grooves (Beau's lines).
- Black nail (runner's toe or tennis toe, a subungual hematoma in which a nailed blackens and eventually falls off)
- Red or purple discoloration (purpura of the nail bed)
- Vertical lines and ridges
- General dryness, splitting and chipping
- Unusual sensitivity
- Faster or slower rate of growth

Sometimes there are more serious side which require the help of a dermatologist:

- Fungal infection (onychomycosis). Nails will thicken and flake.
- Yeast infection. Nails will turn yellow, brown, or white. It is important to treat this immediately, as the infection can spread to the mouth.
- Paronychia. A bacterial or fungal infection that causes inflammation to at the base of the nails.
- Green nails (pseudomonas). A bacterial infection that happens when the nail bed is lifted and bacteria enters under the nail plate or, in the case of acrylic nails, between the natural and artificial nail.

Many of these changes can be helped from a cosmetic and comfort standpoint, but it is important to take nail care seriously during cancer treatment. Cuticle tearing, hangnails, cuts, and other injuries can put you at the risk for infection. If you had lymph node dissection as part of breast surgery, you should be extra careful not to damage your nails. Moisturizing and protecting nails is very important too, for reasons of comfort as well as looks. Nail changes will go away after treatment, usually within six months, and your nails will grow out normally.

Here are some general guidelines to nail health during treatment:

- Keep nails neatly trimmed, and file edges so they are smooth.
- Discontinue use of acrylic nails, silk wraps, glue manicures, and other nail wraps.
- Massage cuticle oil or cream into cuticles to moisturize cuticles and nails and prevent cracking and hangnails.
- Use cuticle remover and gently push back cuticles instead of cutting.
- Do not pick at your nails: brittle or softened nails can lift from the bed and invite infection.
- Switch to a non acetone nail polish remover. Acetone can be drying.
- Avoid prolonged exposure to water, which can lead to a fungal infection.
- Wear nail polish to protect the nails, make them stronger, and discourage picking.
- Drink plenty of fluids to discourage nails from peeling.
- Alert your doctor if you see any inflammation, infection, or unusual changes in your nails.
- Remember to wear sunscreen!

> **NAIL CARE AND LYMPHEDEMA:**
> *Taking good care of your nails during chemotherapy is the first line of defense against lymphedema, in which lymph fluid accumulates in the soft tissues of the arm, causing it to swell. If you've had an underarm lymph node dissection (with mastectomy or lumpectomy), you should be particularly careful of damage to the nail, such as hangnails, cuts, or burns on the hands or fingers, which could lead to infection.*

Here are a few additional suggestions for nail care from Dr. Debra Jaliman:

- Keep your nails hydrated. Rub a small amount of a moisturizing cream into the nail and the cuticle before you go to bed. You can even use petrolatum.

- Protect nails as much as possible during the day: wear cotton-lined gloves when doing the dishes, as this will help protect your nails. Make certain to dry your hands very well when removing the gloves
- Use a superfatted soap or mild cleanser to wash your hands, as detergents soaps can be very harsh and drying.
- Consider wearing nail polish both to protect the nails and hide discoloration: Clinique and Almay both make nail polishes that tend to be less allergic than other brands. Try dark nail polish to hide any discoloration.
- Take 2.5mgs of biotin per day to strengthen your nails. Biotin can increase nail thickness by 22 percent!

A prescription cream called Genadur can help strengthen nails. Use it in the evening, as it washes off during the day.

FREQUENTLY ASKED QUESTIONS ABOUT NAIL CARE

Can I get manicures and pedicures during chemotherapy?
Yes…but very cautiously, and ask your oncology team first. If a salon is not scrupulous about sanitizing, you can get a fungal infection. If your oncologist gives you the go-ahead, here are some tips to help keep you safe:

- Let your nail technician know you are undergoing chemotherapy. Ask her to wash her hands thoroughly before beginning.
- Bring your own set of nail tools, including a rounded cuticle pusher (squared-off ones are too tough).
- Bring your own nontoxic nail polish remover and nail polish. Although you may not think that a salon's nail polishes can harbor bacteria, they can.
- Ask your technician to be extra gentle with your nails, as they may be weakened.
- Avoid soaking in manicure bowls or pedicure tubs. Ask that your nails be massaged with nail oil and allow some time for it to soften the cuticles before pushing them back.

- Do not let her cut cuticles. Ask her to push them back gently with your rounded pusher.
- Much as you may want to, avoid artificial nails, nail wraps, glue manicures, and other nail wraps.

Avoid any aggressive scraping of callouses and especially "Credo" blades used to remove callouses (which really should not be used under any circumstances!).

What chemotherapy drugs cause the most changes in fingernails and toenails?
According to research, the most common are docetaxel (Taxotere), paclitaxel (Taxol), doxorubicin (Adriamycin), epirubicin (Ellence), and capecitabine (Xeloda).

What chemo drug may be causing my nails to soften?
Dr. Noëlle Sherber: "Women receiving paclitaxel may have shedding of their nails. This is the result of UV light interacting with the nails (termed photo-onycholysis), so the best prevention is to keep the nails painted with opaque polish to prevent UV light from contacting them." This can also hide any discoloration you may have.

Is there anything I can do to prevent nail changes?
Maybe through use of a cold cap, which is becoming a common device to preserve hair from loss during chemotherapy. New research shows that cooling hands and nails with ice during chemotherapy treatments may decrease the severity of nail changes. Speak with your oncology team.

Is there a nutritional supplement I can try for nail regrowth?
Possibly. Dr. Alan Bauman has seen improvement in nails by taking the hair regrowth supplement Viviscal.

Nail Care Tips from Survivors

"Chemo made all my nails fall off one by one. As new nails grew in, they didn't know which way to grow, so that produced a lot of ingrown toe nails. I had a good friend who helped me avoid toe nail surgery, as she was a pedicurist. I suggest making friends with someone in that field. My toenails are kept trimmed because they are still brittle. Biotin is a supplement I now take to help my skin and nails. As long as I am on tamoxifen, I am dry-skinned and will have brittle nails and hair. Biotin makes all the different for me." —Lynn Jones

"Using a good-quality cuticle oil (CND Solar Oil or almond oil if you're on a budget) daily regularly massaged into the nail and cuticle helps. Warm a little oil up in a cup and just sit the finger ends in for five minutes, then massage the remainder into your hands." —Cindy Woodward, skin-care therapist at the Beauty Retreat Organic Day Spa, Sheffield, England

"I continued to get manicures and kept my nails short. I bought all my own tools to the salon with me. Keeping my nails up and polished made me feel better when I looked at my hands with the chemo tubes coming out of them. I did lose my big toenails after chemo and keep polish on the remaining eight!" —Aileen Gold

"During chemo…my fingernails were dark. A nurse advised me to use tea tree oil on my nails." —Chris Hart-Wright

"Take good care of your nails. They may fall off during or after chemotherapy. Keep them short and use a good nail hardener. If you develop brown spots on the nail bed *do not* try to file them off. You will damage your nail bed. They may be tender." —Jori Walker

"I sprayed my nails a few times each day with hydrogen peroxide. This prevented spotting on my nails and possibly losing them." —Heidi Bright, M. Div., www.heidibright.com

CHAPTER TWO

HAIR CARE DURING CANCER TREATMENT

HAIR LOSS CAN BE THE MOST dramatic side effect of chemotherapy. Yes, indeed. Five years later, I still cringe at the thought. It took me a while to write an introduction to this chapter. I sat in front of my computer, staring at the blank screen, remembering all the "dramatic" moments of my recovery process that had to do with my hair issues. Before my chemo treatments began, my hair was dark brown and waist long. Some people actually thought I had extensions, but it was all mine! My oncologist said that my chemotherapy was not supposed to cause all of the hair to fall out. She assured me that I should lose no more than 60 percent of my hair. Sixty percent? What in the world is 60 percent of a head full of hair? I had absolutely no idea what to expect. After my second treatment, my dark brown hair turned red; after the third it started to clump, and after the fourth, fall, one hair at a time. If I wore a backless shirt or a tank top, I could actually feel it falling out and down my back. A month *after* my chemo treatments ended, I went to New Orleans with some friends. By that time, I cut my hair to shoulder length and had it layered hoping to minimize the look of thinning hair. In the hotel, my hair began to fall out in big, ugly clumps. I had to sleek it back into a bun and pray that I would make it back to New York without going completely bald. Three days later, I sat in the office of a Park Avenue doctor specializing in hair preservation and restoration, weeping out loud and showing him a picture of what used to be my glorious, waist long hair.

I am almost embarrassed to say it now, but the loss of my hair was almost as painful as my diagnosis. But I am not alone! I did not want for people to know that I was sick, but nothing screams "cancer" as does a bald head or lack of eye brows. For more than 70 percent of women undergoing cancer treatment, hair loss (also referred to as *alopecia*) is inevitable. Even though, hair loss is usually temporary and hair will grow back, it is no less devastating. It may also take up to a year for hair to be the state that will make you happy.

The purpose of this chapter as well as the whole *Surviving Beautifully* project is to identify aesthetic issues and to show you solutions that will either eliminate or at least help you deal with these issues successfully. Many groundbreaking medical methods could have helped me reduce my hair loss if I had just known about them. If I had planned better, I would have saved myself a lot of emotional pain. It's terrible to know that the control has been whisked from you, and we want to show you ways to take it back. In this chapter, we will discuss these issues:

- The effects of chemotherapy, radiation, and hormone therapy on hair
- Stages of hair thinning or hair release (Notice that throughout this chapter we refer to the process of losing your hair as *hair release*. Using the word *release* provides a gentle reminder that for most people this is a *temporary* stage of the healing process that shall pass.)
- Understanding percentages of hair release and what it means visually. Many new cancer treatments do not cause full loss of hair. Understanding how much hair you may lose and what it will look like can help you with decision making.
- Methods of slowing down hair release or even stopping it all together
- Preparing yourself emotionally for hair release
- If saving hair is not a possibility in your case, we will discuss the choices:
- caring for scalp and for thinning hair
- caring for scalp if you choose the bald look
- preparing for wearing a wig, wig types and alternatives, caring for wigs

- other head cover options
- hair after cancer treatments
- brows and lashes

This chapter will provide you with choices and give you a timeline of hair release and regrowth. One of the reasons that hair may fall out is emotional stress. However, if you prepare yourself, you can minimize this stress significantly. You will see that you do not have to spend a lot of money to look like yourself with a wig that replicates your style. Or you may choose to have fun experimenting with new looks. Many modern options are available to you if in rare case your hair does not rebound as well as you would like. Although we do not discuss nutrition in this book, a healthy diet is key to good hair and skin.

As for me, my hair did grow back fully. It did not fall out completely, but I cut it short and wore a wig because I could not color my hair and did not want to show gray. I got tons of compliments on my new hairdo and my bravery in experimenting with new styles. I wound up liking my short cut so much that I wore it for a long time in full curls like Marilyn Monroe. The trick is to see this time of your life as a challenge, not as torture. You will be surprised that you may even have fun.

WHY HAIR RELEASES
Chemotherapy

Chemotherapy attacks rapidly growing cancer cells. Like the cells in the skin, hair cells also rapidly grow and divide and are therefore prone to changes. Although your skin and mouth may change in any number of ways, hair almost universally behaves the same: it simply releases. This includes eyebrows and eyelashes, hair on your body, and pubic hair. Fortunately, this is almost always temporary.

As with every chemotherapy treatment, some drugs or combinations of drugs are more likely to cause hair release. Occasionally, some will result in permanent hair loss. Here are some general guidelines—always check with your oncology team for more specific information. No two patients are alike.

Radiation

Radiation usually does not cause hair release, and if it does, it is only in the area being treated. For example, if you're getting radiation to your head, hair is likely to release only where the beam is aimed—and maybe eyebrows and eyelashes too. If you're getting radiation treatment on other areas of the body (like for breast or ovarian cancer), hair local to that part of the body may release (hair around nipple, under the arms, or the pubic region).

However radiation can cause more problems with hair regrowth. Changes in hair regrowth from radiation damage can be permanent, and hair can grow back in patches, be thinner, or have a different texture. For some women, this is a silver lining: a woman with fine hair may come out of her treatment with a thick head of curls; at the same time, hair can regrow in different colors or be prematurely gray.

Tamoxifen or Other Hormone Therapy

The effects of hormone treatment like tamoxifen on hair are much less universal than those from chemotherapy or radiation. Because it suppresses the production of estrogen, which can accelerate and improve hair growth (as during pregnancy), tamoxifen can drive hair follicles to remain in a resting state, thus not grow. Many women on tamoxifen experience hair thinning despite the medical literature that claims that only a 1 to 5 percent of women experience this side effect. This can be the most distressing part of long-term or preventative cancer treatment: most people expect hair release during cancer treatment, to endure it for years *afterwards* adds insult to injury. However, as with chemo and radiation, there are many alternatives to cope with hair release, short or long term.

STAGES OF HAIR RELEASE

If you are having chemotherapy...

Before beginning treatment, consult with your oncologist and review your chemo cocktail. Different drugs have different effects on hair, and your oncologist can give you an idea of what you might expect. Based on this info, you can begin thinking about how to prepare for complete hair release, if it should happen. If you plan to wear a head covering, *this is the time to decide what is right for you!*

Hairpieces, wigs, and other hair prosthetics may be covered under your insurance plan. Some insurance companies will pay for a wig, also called a medical prosthesis or prosthetic or durable medical equipment (DME), and your doctor will write a prescription for one just as he or she would for any other medication.

However, for many women, health insurance coverage has limited benefits, according to independent insurance agent (and breast cancer survivor) Kristy Fishman. She says that insurance plans pay for a percentage, but the following may apply before you receive the benefits:

- *Your deductible has been met, out of pocket maximum has been met*
- *The wig provider is a participating provider or in-network provider*
- *The plan may only pay for one wig up to a maximum dollar amount*
- *If your plan allows, submit a claim form along with the receipt and a prescription from your doctor. The prescription should include the diagnosis code (very important), otherwise your claim may not be paid. Note: some wig providers offer discounts to patients receiving chemotherapy. If they do not offer this to you, ask.*
- *Additionally, any head coverings you pay for out of pocket may be tax deductible as medical expenses. Check with your accountant to be sure.*
- *If you do not have insurance or your insurance company will not pay for a wig, contact your local branch of the American Cancer Society or other cancer support organizations, which often provide wigs donated by women who have recovered from cancer.*

Hair changes may occur at the very start of chemotherapy, with hair becoming drier and more brittle. But hair release usually begins between one and three weeks after chemo. Hair can release gradually or literally in clumps depending on the drug. For example, Adriamycin causes hair to fall out gradually, but Taxol often causes hair to fall out suddenly. Consult our chart in the Appendix for more details.

Hair thinning and release continues during the course of your treatment.

About three weeks after treatment ends, hair regrowth will begin. It will likely be very downy, like baby hair. Hair texture may be different at first (or permanently).

About six months to a year after completing treatment, hair should regrow normally.

If you are getting radiation...

Hair release usually begins two to three weeks after your first treatment. Remember, you will only lose hair at the site of radiation!

Hair release from radiation is quick: it usually takes only about a week. You may notice your newly exposed skin is tender or inflamed, like a sunburn. If you had radiation to your head, your scalp and eyebrow/eyelash areas may be dry and irritated. See your dermatologist. Hair regrowth usually begins three to six months after treatment ends. Hair texture may be different at first.

NEW TREATMENTS THAT MAY SLOW HAIR RELEASE

Hair release is such a prevalent issue during cancer treatment that the medical community is always searching for ways to minimize "looking sick." Here are some promising options you may wish to discuss with your oncology team.

Scalp Hypothermia or Cryotherapy

Simply put, keeping the head cold during the administration of chemotherapy can slow or even prevent hair release. This is usually done with a "cold cap," a soft helmet-like hat filled with gel that is frozen before use. It is purchased or rented by the patient and is worn before, during, and for a short while after chemotherapy sessions. It freezes the scalp and hair follicles so that chemotherapy drugs do not reach, and therefore damage, hair follicles. Caps may be changed during use to keep them very cold.

Many women report they kept their hair using a cold cap, while others report their hair thinned, rather than completely released. In fact, up to 73 percent of women using a cold cap kept their hair! British studies show that success can be up to 85 percent with certain chemotherapy drugs such as Taxotere, Taxol, epirubicin, and Cyclophosphamide.

The drawback to using this device—in which you may have to invest in coolers as well as renting the cap itself—is that it is costly (up to $5,000) and may not be covered by insurance. A few cold cap assistance programs have been created to help defray the cost, including Rapunzel Project (www.rapunzelproject.org) and CCAPS (www.ccaps.org).

Although cold caps may be a great option to preserve hair, they may not be right for people receiving strong doses of chemotherapy, if you're having chemotherapy for prolonged periods of time through a pump, or if you suffer from migraines. They can be heavy and uncomfortable. Furthermore, they will not preserve hair on other parts of your body, including eyebrows and eyelashes.

Laser Cap Treatment

Dr. Alan Bauman of the Bauman Medical Group has found that low-level light therapy (LLLT) may stimulate and increase blood supply to the scalp and preserve hair follicles, therefore slowing hair release. Some studies show that it is effective in up to 85 percent of patients. LLLT is administered through a laser cap, a portable low-dose laser therapy device worn on the head. Treatment is administered for thirty minutes, two to three times a week for about eight or nine weeks. The treatment is not painful, although some patients report tingling. As with a cold cap, LLLT treatment may not be covered by insurance and the treatments may be costly. They are found to be particularly effective to restore regrowth *after* treatment or for permanent thinning or alopecia.

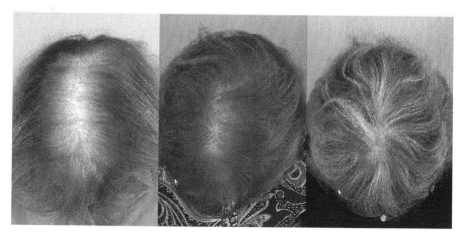

Laser cap treatment before, 6 months, and 12 months
after chemotherapy, by Dr. Alan J. Bauman

TOPICAL TREATMENTS

Minoxidil

Minoxidil (Rogaine) is an FDA-approved drug to treat male-pattern baldness in both men and women. It *might* delay hair release during chemotherapy and shorten its duration, according to the Mayo Clinic, but will not prevent it., and the results are inconclusive. However, it may be something to look into, and it certainly has been proven to help with hair regrowth in men.

Minoxidil is usually applied twice daily during your chemotherapy treatment and for four months afterward. Dr. Bauman notes: "OTC minoxidil is not as effective and has more side-effects than the prescription (Formula 82M) versions." The drawbacks are the cost and possible scalp irritation. If you do try minoxidil, be sure not to apply it anywhere you don't want hair to grow!

Note: there is now Women's Rogaine, which may also help regrow hair; it may also reverse the progression of hereditary baldness.

ThymuSkin

ThymuSkin is a line of topical treatments based on the thymus gland, an organ in the chest involved with developing white blood cells. It was developed in Germany to treat a variety of scalp issues and alopecia and comes in the form of shampoos and gels that, according to a double-blind clinical trial by doctors in Europe, can help prevent hair loss during chemotherapy treatment. It seems to work best for patients who are treated with 5-FU rather than Adriamycin. Results are mixed, but Internet reviews are more or less positive. The downside is the cost: over $100 for the starter kit.

WHAT DOES 25, 50, OR 75 PERCENT HAIR LOSS LOOK LIKE?

During chemotherapy, your hair is put into, and *stays*, in its resting phase known as *telogen*, states hair replacement expert Lucinda Ellery. Telogen happens to us every day regardless of medical treatment. An average head has up to 150,000 healthy hairs and sheds 50 to 125 of these a day. However, during chemo the hair follicles remain dormant until treatment is completed. Thus, no new hair grows in to replace hair that has shed. Loss starts becoming visible when more than a hundred hairs come out regularly.

Hair release from chemotherapy and radiation usually takes the form of female pattern baldness. Dr. Alan Bauman explains: "Hair loss looks different in women than men. Hair loss in men causes a receding hairline and loss of coverage in the crown/vertex area. In women, the hairline typically does not change, but they lose density…in [the] frontal area first, then it can progress to the crown."

Doctors often talk about hair release in terms of figures like "50 percent" hair loss, which can be hard for patients to comprehend. Dr. Bauman clarifies: "It's hard for patients to imagine 10–50 percent loss because it's hard to 'see.' Studies have been done which show that if you physically remove 50 percent of the hair fibers from a given area of scalp, it looks *exactly* the same. Now, obviously, it doesn't feel or behave the same. That is why we (hair doctors) say that you can lose up to 50 percent of your hair without it being noticeable to the naked eye. If the average person drops below 50 percent density, that's when it starts to look thin to the naked eye and styling becomes a challenge." But, he adds, the "'reality' is that women don't just lose density…they also experience a loss of hair caliber," that is, mass. So not only might you have less hair, you may have thinner hair too.

PREPARING YOURSELF FOR HAIR RELEASE

Emotionally preparing yourself is very important to managing chemotherapy- and radiation-induced hair release, but here are some practical tips as well:

- Have some good-quality images taken of your hair at its best. Take close-up as well as portrait shots in natural light. You can use these later to help match the color of your wig. They are also a great reference point for your hairdresser to use to style your hair when it grows back in.
- Purchase lightweight cotton stretch caps and warm fleece hats now. You may want to use them to prevent chills during chemotherapy as well as to regulate your body heat in general.

- Invest in satin or silk pillowcases. These will reduce tangling while hair releases and feel better on the scalp.
- Get in the habit of treating your hair and scalp gently *now*. The more gentle you are on your hair, the longer it will stick around.

HAIR AND SCALP CARE BEFORE TREATMENT

Although you may not be able to do anything to prevent hair release entirely, you can take many actions *before* your treatment begins or if you experience just hair thinning. These simple steps can help your hair and scalp be in the best condition to prevent further loss.

- Make sure your hair is clean and free of tangles and products. Do not brush, manipulate, or scratch the scalp before starting treatment, as this can invite infection, according to hair expert Toni Love.
- Use conditioner to make combing wet hair easier, and comb and brush hair gently: a wide-toothed comb can help.
- Stop using very hot blow dryers, flatirons, curling irons, or other devices that put stress on hair and scalp.
- Lay off chemical treatments for hair six to eight weeks before chemotherapy begins. Hair expert Toni Love says: "There should not be any chemicals (color, relaxer, permanent waves, bleach) applied to the hair...these will weaken the hair, resulting in rapid hair loss. Not every woman loses all of her hair as she undergoes chemotherapy, especially if the hair is 'virgin' and free of chemicals."
- Avoid braiding, tight ponytails, or other hairstyles that pull at the scalp.
- If you have long hair, invest in a silk hair net to wear while sleeping. This contains the hair and discourages tangling and strain on the scalp.
- Avoid heavy-duty styling products that "stick" in the hair and require more aggressive washing or extra shampoo to wash out.
- Stop dyeing hair or getting perms.

- While hair is thinning, use a volumizing shampoo and "soft hold" volumizing product to give it a thicker feel.
- Consider cutting your hair now! Not only will it ease the stress if hair starts releasing drastically, it can minimize the appearance of thinning. And doing so may help you—and others—prepare for further release. See below.
- Stop using rubber bathing caps if you swim regularly. A smooth Lycra one may be a better choice.
- Very important! Find a *professional hair loss expert*. She can help guide you through the stages of hair loss and help you choose the best options for head coverings during treatment as well as post treatment care.

SCALP CARE DURING CANCER TREATMENT

You may find that your hair is temporarily gone and your scalp is now exposed, perhaps for the first time ever, and you may experience scalp sensitivity. Here are tips on how to minimize discomfort from hair release and promote scalp health for future regrowth.

- Baby the scalp. Now that you no longer have hair, it's no longer necessary to shampoo it! Try using a gentle facial cleanser instead, and pat—don't rub—your scalp dry. Vigorous rubbing can irritate your scalp.
- Replace hair conditioner with a moisturizer because chemotherapy may dry your scalp in the same way it does the rest of your body. You can use facial moisturizer.
- Resist the temptation to use bar soap on your head.
- Consider shaving your head if you have annoying, itchy stubble or patchiness.
- Use a chemical free, high-SPF sunscreen to protect the naked scalp. See our Appendix for suggestions.
- If you get scalp acne, treat in the same way as your face (see our Skin Care chapter).

- If you have dry skin, try a natural oil like olive, Vitamin E or olive oil to calm and help reestablish the protective oil layer. You can add lavender and chamomile soothe, or lemon oil for dryness and flaking. Rosemary and peppermint stimulate growth by increasing microcirculation. Some hair dressers like Phyto Phytopolleine Scalp Stimulant: one bottle contains an effective blend of essential oils that stimulate circulation, soothe inflammation, and balance.
- Carry baby wipes with you to freshen your scalp during the day, particularly after you exercise.
- If you lose underarm hair, you may experience irritation and sensitivity there too. Switch to a natural deodorant and moisturizer, if necessary.
- Be sure to see your doctor if you experience sores, significant itching or flakiness, or a rash.

HAIR CARE FOR THINNING HAIR

Most survivors experience hair thinning and brittleness even if the hair does not release entirely. Lola Bennett, hairstylist at Yves Durif Salon at the Carlyle, suggests you start at the root of it all: "I always emphasize the importance of good scalp care to people with weak or thinning hair. Each hair comes through an opening in the scalp called the follicle. The follicle influences the shape and size of the hair, and if the follicle is too small the hair trying to come through will be much smaller in diameter than it should be. The best way to keep the scalp healthy is to use care when styling; hairstyles that are too tight can lead to breakage, hair loss, or inflammation." Here are some more tips to encourage health and growth:

- Do gentle scalp massage and brushing. It's extremely important to use only a high-quality, gentle brush. Take great care when brushing hair from scalp to ends, as brushing too vigorously can cause scalp abrasions and exacerbate any existing conditions. Natural bristles are best.
- Shampoo as little as possible.

- Weekly deep-conditioning treatments are also great for dryness and flaking. To do a deep condition, shampoo hair and apply a rich conditioner all over, wrap hair in a damp, warm towel, process for fifteen minutes, and rinse thoroughly.
- Celebrity colorist Corey Powell recommends stimulating the scalp by brushing with a Mason-Pearson natural brush and using Rene Furterer Complexe 5 or tea tree oil.
- Switch to a volumizing shampoo: Dr. Alan Bauman likes Pantene AgeDefy Hair Thickening. "Consistent daily use makes your hair measurably thicker and fuller, feel healthier and improves coverage of the scalp. It works by smoothly coating each individual hair strand making your hair 'perform' better, requiring less styling effort."
- Minoxidil or Nioxin shampoo may help retain existing hair and improve hair regrowth.

> *When you are in full stages of hair release, consider putting a towel over your pillow to make morning clean-up easier.*

WHEN FIRST TO CUT YOUR HAIR

Most doctors, websites, and survivors suggest cutting hair short or shaving it entirely *before* hair release begins to get the trauma over with. Hairdresser Isaac Mann puts is succinctly: "Why torture yourself with seeing your hair fall out every day? It just adds more stress." Don't let cancer boss you around: if you deal with the inevitable as soon as possible, you will feel you have more control.

But is this right for you? Some people think this will make the transition easier, while other experts suggest when your hair releases, you go right into wearing a wig that closely resembles your own hair with no intermediary step. The choice is yours.

Think about cutting your hair if the following conditions apply to you:

- Your hair has already changed in texture and thinned from chemotherapy even though it hasn't released entirely.

- You do not want to wear a wig and want to prep yourself, your family, coworkers, and friends for "a new you."
- You color or process your hair and can't continue during treatment, but don't want to wear a wig.
- Short hair release "feels" easier to manage than long hair release.
- You've been thinking about experimenting with a new style anyway: you can then "spin" your new look into a personal choice.

If you do decide to cut your hair, have a discussion with your hairdresser to let him or her know what is going on. Your hairdresser can plan your new cut appropriately to make the most of your hair and be easier to style if your hair starts thinning. He or she will also have tips to help disguise thinning hair and keep it in the best condition.

If you don't want to transition from your hair to short hair to (maybe) no hair, *or* plan to have a wig fitted or wear a head covering as soon as possible after diagnosis, then shaving your head preemptively may be right for you.

Rather than just grab an old razor or electric hair clippers and have at it, take a few moments to pamper yourself and get your scalp off to a good start. Buy a high-quality razor (some pros recommend Gillette Mach 3 razors, and others those with a flexible head. Ask a male friend!), get a friend to help, enjoy a glass of wine, and think of this as one a one step closer to healing.

- Clip or cut hair to a quarter inch at most.
- Get in the shower and *thoroughly* wet your head. Exfoliate your scalp with a gentle scrub. This not only softens the hair but lifts the hair to reduce the chance of "razor burn" or ingrown hairs.
- *Generously* apply a shaving lubricant. You can use the same type made for either the face or legs.
- Begin with the front of your head, where hair is softer. Shave with the grain of hair from the top of the head down the sides, gently. Then back to front. Don't apply pressure!

- When you're done, give your head a nice cool rinse to close pores. Apply a natural aftershave cream.

WIGS AND HAIRPIECES

Many women opt to wear wigs during chemotherapy, and good, natural-looking wigs are now available in all price ranges. Wigs are no longer one solid color, and the synthetic hair is no longer as detectable. The trick it to find one that looks as much as possible like you.

Most experts agree that you should go to a wig salon *before* you begin your chemotherapy/radiation treatments, "with your image intact, so we can see the texture and the cut," adds Barry Hendrickson, owner of Bitz-n-Pieces in Manhattan and author of *Looking Like You: A Step-by-Step Guide for Medical Hair Replacement.* "You will still look like your old self, and your hair stylist will be able to create a look that is similar." Going to a salon early also gives you and your wig stylist time to prepare and have your wig ready as soon as you need it. So book an appointment at a wig salon before your hair releases and while you still have energy. Having a beautiful, natural wig waiting in the wings for you can ease your mind and help you relax. You will feel more secure knowing that you have a solution for when your hair does release, whether it goes slowly or overnight.

It is very important to work with a professional wig salon rather than order one in a catalog or on the Internet that you can't try on. Wig specialists are attuned to the stress you are going through and privacy you desire, and they will gently guide you through the process, be respectful of your price range, and help you get the best look for you. Finding a pro can make all the difference between wearing a beautiful, "invisible," and comfortable wig versus an ill-fitting, painful, and obvious wig. Your hospital or support group may have local referrals.

Because the emotional impact of hair releasing can be so strong, many women find it very valuable to maintain their current look. For these women, now is not the time for a complete change. "Looking like you is very important at this time…finding the delicate balance between facing reality and creating it can work miracles in healing," states Barry Hendrickson. This is particularly important if you want to keep your treatments private.

If you want to ease the transition and wear a wig undetected, here is a simple step-by-step timeline:

1. Educate yourself about the types of wigs that are available (see below).
2. Call your health insurance company. Find out what they need from your doctor to submit a claim, and find out how much they will cover! This will help you set a price point for your wig and avoid wasted time and disappointment in looking at wigs out of your price range.
3. Get a prescription from your oncologist for a wig. Ask your insurance company the exact phrase you should use to get it covered.
4. At the same time, find out what kind of paperwork from the *wig salon* your insurance company will want you to submit with your claim. Your salon may need to write an invoice in a specific way. Better to know now.
5. Have a consultation with a wig master. Once you have your appointment made, gather things to bring to the salon. This should include a photo of you in your usual hairstyle (one that you like) and images from magazines or the Internet of styles you like. While most people stress the importance of not dramatically changing your look right now, you may want to be open to possibilities. For example, if you currently have long hair, you may resist getting a shorter wig; however, this may be easier to care for and style than a long wig when you're in the midst of exhausting chemotherapy treatments or after surgery.

Start by trying on wigs, but do not have a wig fitting at your first appointment. There is no point to fitting a wig on a full head of hair when you will not have that hair soon. The wig will fit poorly and be uncomfortable. The last thing you want is for your wig to be an ordeal too.

It is up to you if you want to bring a friend or family member to the wig salon with you. Friends and family mean well, but they also bring with them their own biases. Our advice is to stick to *one* friend/family member at most. The process of choosing a wig is very personal and emotional. Having too many people weighing in can confuse you and add to the stress.

6. Once your hair releases, go back for your wig fitting. At the fitting, discuss the care of your wig, strategies for wearing it without detection, styling at home, and a schedule for any future professional styling that may be needed.

Types of Wigs

We suggest you determine a price range before shopping for a wig to help narrow choices and put you in control. If your budget is five hundred dollars out of pocket, there is no reason to spend a lot of time looking at four thousand dollar wigs and getting depressed. However, it may be worth it to stretch your budget *a little* to get the best look for you that will make you *feel* better about your looks and treatment. Your wig salon will guide you.

There are two categories of wigs: ready-to-wear and custom-made. Within each category are several types: synthetic, a blend of synthetic and human hair (called "human hair blends"), and natural human hair. Synthetic and human hair blend wigs can be either ready-to-wear or custom-made. Human hair wigs are most often custom-made.

The way a wig is constructed will be a big factor in how it looks, moves, and behaves. There are three types: machine-made, hand-made, and custom-made. Machine-made wigs have wefts of hair sewn in a straight line, cut and assembled to look like a wig. They are widely available and tend to be inexpensive. With the right styling, they actually *can* be realistic. Hand-made wigs have the hair wefts individually knotted into a nylon mesh. They can be worn parted and, because the hair is individually knotted, tend to move more naturally. Custom-made wigs are the gold standard in natural look and feel. They can barely be distinguished from natural hair. This look comes at a price, though: they can be two thousand dollars and up and take months to complete.

Synthetic Wigs

Don't shy away from the word *synthetic*. Synthetic wigs have come a long way from the heavy, unnatural ones of the past and can be quite natural in texture and color. Wig master Isaac Davidson explains: "The hair now does not have the fake shine of synthetic hair of the past. You can also style the new synthetics with heat, just like natural hair." Another benefit of synthetic wigs is that they keep their style when it is humid and hold the style better in general.

Keep in mind that an inexpensive wig may look fine, but if the fibers are seated on a thick nylon cap, it can be virtually unwearable and cause scalp problems to boot. Be sure to examine the wig from beneath: you should be able to see through the cap. Only choose wigs with natural liners like silk, advises hair loss expert Elline Surianello. This indicates your scalp will be able to breathe and the wig will feel light. Synthetic wigs usually cost between forty and five hundred dollars.

> **PURCHASE MORE THAN ONE WIG.**
> *If you can, have a fresh backup wig at all times. Many women purchase a more expensive natural or blend wig, and an inexpensive synthetic one to wear at the gym or at home. Cancer survivor Harriet notes: "There is enormous comfort and reassurance in having (and also sometimes carrying with you) more than one wig, especially for those of us who travel and/or continue to work during treatment. Then, as unexpected incidents arise—sudden rain downpours, high winds, as happened to me walking on bridge across the Chicago River with wig ending up in the water, lost luggage—the worry about showing up bald or disheveled does not create incremental agita to the underriding concern about being bald."*

Synthetic and Human Hair Blends

Wigmakers know there is real value in natural-looking but easy-to-maintain wigs, and the new crop of synthetic and human hair blend wigs reflects this. These wigs are gaining in popularity because they offer a more natural look with the easy, versatile styling and upkeep of synthetic fibers. Hair expert Toni Love notes: "Blended wigs are a great choice for those wanting the feel of human hair and who want the style to last longer without the daily maintenance of a human hair wig. The blended wigs require low to no heat when styling, since the synthetic hair is made out of a fiber."

Human Hair

Wigs made from human hair naturally will look most like real hair. You can style them as you would your natural hair, and they often have a super-light cap, offering the greatest comfort. Human hair is usually Asian or European. Asian hair is thicker and stronger, but can also be coarser. European hair is more expensive but has greater natural wave and sheen. As with any custom-made wig, human hair wigs are expensive (about three thousand five hundred dollars and up) and require more maintenance.

A final consideration is a wig *cap* itself. You may or may not want to wear one if your hair has entirely released; if you do have hair, however, you will have to for the wig to fit correctly. Experts agree that a very lightweight mesh, lace, or gauzy "monofilament" cap is best.

We suggest you go for the best wig you can afford and plan to have it *professionally styled after it is fitted*. A stylist's attention to detail and personal touches like highlights or layers can mean all the difference in how natural the wig may look. It's worth it: a nicely styled wig can really lift your spirits and keep you positive during your healing journey.

Wig salons are now offering a new way to look like you during treatment by creating a custom wig out of your own hair which is cut before it releases. One advantage to this procedure is that the wig will be very natural looking and virtually undetectable. Another plus is that you already know how to style the hair. Additional hair may be needed to fill out the wig, and you will still have the same issues in caring for it as you would human hair. Prices are about two thousand dollars and up.

Choosing the Most Natural Color and Style for You

Most experts advise you to match your wig to your natural hair as much as possible, however, do keep a few things in mind:

- You may want to choose a color lighter than your natural hair. Skin may take on a yellowish or grayish cast from chemotherapy, therefore increasing the contrast with your hair. Hair expert Lucinda Ellery explains: "Wigs look more natural if they are one shade lighter than your own hair color, as your skin tone does change while undergoing any intensive medical treatment." Furthermore, your wig hair may be thicker than your own hair: dark colors will only highlight this more and reveal that your "hair" may not be natural.

- Consider a shorter wig even if you have long hair: it may be easier to care for.

- If you choose to go with a different color wig, consider your eyebrows. Don't go too light if you have dark eyebrows as it will look unnatural. You can always darken light brows, but it's very hard to lighten dark brows.

> We know wigs can help with the emotional pain of losing your hair during cancer treatment… but physical pain too? Linda Ellery relays this story: "A wig can definitely help, not only with aesthetics but also with pain management! I once visited a patient in hospital who would not allow anyone to touch her hair, but she was in a lot of pain as the lost hair had become entangled with the hair that was still securely anchored within the follicles. I spent an hour or more listening to her concerns. The main one was that she felt if her hair was cut, she would never have it back and she would not feel feminine. I explained that she would feel more comfortable and there would be less chance of infection if the hairs that were under tension were removed. She agreed and I cut away the matted hair and fitted a wig, which was then cut and styled to suit her. A few months later, the lady came to see me. Her hair had regrown, and she said that it had really helped to discuss her fears and that the wig helped her through this not only physically but also emotionally difficult period in her life."

- If your hair has not fully released and is fairly close to your wig color, you can try blending in your own hair along the hairline for a more natural look. Apply your wig, and then pull out small sections of your own hair along the sides and front using your fingers or a rattail comb.
- Don't overhandle your wig: a little hand fluffing may be all you need if your wig is prestyled.

Wearing Your New Wig

Wearing a wig might take a bit of getting used to. In addition to having a sensitive scalp, you will now have something "foreign" on your head. You may be nervous it will slip, fall off, or otherwise move. Here are some tips to help you wear your wig comfortably and keep it secure:

- Wear your wig for short periods of time during the first few days to get used to the feel of it and how it moves.
- Resist the urge to play with and fuss with your wig: doing this looks unnatural and draws attention to it.
- Try not to worry about it falling off. Many wigs are fitted with elastic bands and clips to secure them. See other suggestions below.
- Do not perfume your wig.
- If your wig is uncomfortable, hair replacement expert Helen Owens notes: "Store-bought wigs are typically made with a track back and lace top, which can irritate the scalp... But if there's an affordability issue, a professional can refer you to a wig store that carries a wig with a lighter material that's more scalp friendly and more reasonable in cost."

Banish Wig Worries

Many women feel much better wearing a wig, but worry that it may fall off or that they don't know how to care for it. Not to worry: today's wigs are very secure and easy to care for. With some added "protection," you can feel confident in almost any situation. Here are some products our experts suggest to give you added security:

- TopStick: a favorite of many wigmakers and stylists
- Sock glue: also referred to as "body adherent," or "garment adhesive," and is widely used by celebrities and models to keep body-baring red carpet gowns in place. Janet Crain says: "My wig fit great. [But] I was in a restaurant in a booth and the person at the booth next to me pulled her jacket and it displace my wig... Then I found sock glue designed to hold up men's socks. I put it on my wig and never was embarrassed again."
- Look for a wig with a rubber lining around the hairline. These offer a tight and secure fit.
- Most importantly, make sure you have your wig fitted *after* your hair releases. As mentioned before, it will fit quite differently if you have it fitted while you still have hair and will be loose, uncomfortable, and potentially irritating once the hair is gone.

Styling and Storage

You must buy a few things to help care for your wig. Couture wig master Isaac Davidson recommends the following basics for storage, style, and care. You might want to have:

- a canvas wig head (for styling)
- a Styrofoam wig head (for storage only: Isaac says they're a "disaster" for styling)
- wig pins
- table clamp

Basic Care

- Try to wash wigs infrequently—once a week is ideal.
- For synthetic wigs, use a clarifying shampoo like Paul Mitchell Tea Tree Special Shampoo. "Synthetic hair build up is different than human, and this gets it nice and clean." Follow this with his recommendation of Pantene Pro-V Daily Moisture Renewal Conditioner for All Hair Types.

- For washing and conditioning human hair wigs, experts agree using a sulfate-free shampoo is best. Isaac likes Pantene Pro-V Daily Moisture Renewal Conditioner for All Hair Types: "This keeps the hair silky. Use only on the ends to avoid weighing hair down. I do NOT recommend the use of all-natural hair products on human hair wigs. The hair does not have your natural oils, making natural products react differently. In fact, they can actually dry the hair out."

Style Tips
- Wash at night: "Wash human or synthetic wigs before bed. Towel dry, and then place on the canvas head. Use a wig pin in each temple and two at the nape, and comb out straight following the desired part. Let the wig dry overnight. This avoids more wear and tear from a blow dryer. In the morning, you can use your styling tools or just a light blow dry to create volume."
- Use low-heat appliances on synthetic hair and keep it to 300 degrees or less. (Note: not all synthetic hair may be styled with heat. Ask your wig master.)

Bad Hair…Behavior

No matter how great your wig is, how realistic (or trendy/fun) it may be, or how comfortable you feel about revealing your treatment, you will inevitably run into people who have bad hair etiquette. Surviving Beautifully founder Lana Koifman says: "In life, there will always be rude people, inappropriate questions, and other embarrassing situations. However, this is the time you take care of yourself and put yourself first." Here are some true experiences Lana had, and how she handled them.

- Situation: someone inappropriately touches your wig.

Lana: "Someone did try to pull on my wig. If someone is trying to touch it, simply gently push their hand away and say 'I am sorry, but you are being rude,' or 'You are acting inappropriately and invading my space.' You do *not* owe anyone any explanation."

- Situation: someone asks if you're wearing a wig.

Lana: "There are a couple of ways to handle this. If you do not want to say you are going through chemo, you can say: 'Yes, I am wearing a wig. I am trying out new hairstyles and maybe even new hair colors.' Or, if they really insist that you are, simply say 'With all due respect, you are being rude. I do not believe I owe anyone an explanation.'"

"If you do not want a long conversation with lots of disclosure about the specifics of your treatment, you can simply say, 'I am going through a healing process after a health scare.' For your own sake, put a positive prospective on things."

- Situation: Someone comments about how great your natural hair was.

Lana: "Yes, I heard 'why did you cut it? Your hair was so beautiful!' You can simply say: 'One thing that I learned about life is that it always changes, and I am trying new things.'"

Other Hair Covering Options

There are many other attractive choices for hair coverings if you don't want to wear a wig, need a break from one, or just want other options. Hair coverings usually take the form of scarves, elegant hair wraps, turbans, and hats. Here are the basics to keep looking great without a wig.

Head Scarves

Whether you wear a wig or not, you will definitely want to invest in a few different scarves. Not only do they provide a break if you're wearing a wig, they can make fashion statements with colorful prints and up-to-the-minute color palettes. We recommend getting traditional and/or head scarves in both an elegant material like silk or satin and cotton. Cotton ones are great for when you're exercising, when it's hot out, or when you want to give your scalp a chance to breathe…but not expose it entirely.

Traditional thirty-five- to thirty-six-inch square scarves are often offered by designers as part of their regular lines. These are not usually marketed to cancer fighters but can be worn in many ways with a little help from videos, and they will double as pretty accessories long after your healing journey. Longer head scarves have more versatility and can be used to protect your neck as well.

- Buy a few scarves in both silk and cotton: silk is more formal but requires more care, whereas cotton can elegant too, and will be easier to maintain.
- Prints may be more flattering than solids.
- Treat yourself…or have your friends and family treat you! Comedian Jenny Saldaña amassed a collection of high-end scarves as gifts during treatment, including Hermes, Pucci, and Chanel. While a Chanel bag may be out of the question, a Chanel scarf is much less expensive…and equally long lasting with the right care.
- A bandana, done right, doesn't need to have a biker style. Buy a few in "alternative" colors like peach, olive, light blue, or soft yellow. Tie them at your nape or at the top of your head for a retro look.
- Your local vintage stores and consignment shops will often have beautiful couture scarves at incredible deals. Have any scarf organically dry-cleaned or hand wash before wearing.

Head Wraps

Head wraps are specialty coverings made for ease and comfort. Most have "tails" at the end to tie easily. They come in a beautiful variety of fabrics, prints, and colors. Here are a few lesser-known options to try out:

- Head wraps with padded fronts give you a little fullness at the hairline.
- Pre-tied head wraps are great for days when you are just exhausted.

director of the Robert H. Robert H. Lurie Comprehensive Cancer Center's Dermatologic Care Center at Northwestern University in Chicago. "These [causes] may include treatment-induced low levels of zinc or iron, thyroid problems, or stress." Tamoxifen can cause hair thinning that continues for the duration of its use, and very rarely aggressive chemotherapy can cause permanent hair loss.

Hair regrowth is a very personal thing: for some women, hair comes back very quickly, whereas others may take months. Many women report that their hair is quite different in texture when it comes back in: wiry, thin, fuzzy, maybe gray or white. It may be patchy or thicker in some areas than other. Dark "chemo curls" are consistently noted too. Curls are thought to be a result of the chemotherapy still in your system after treatment, which takes some time to flush out...but the truth is that no one really knows. These changes may be displeasing, and many women opt to continue wearing a wig until their hair returns in its more normal form.

When hair begins to regrow, your focus must be on maintaining scalp health and encouraging growth. Be gentle to your new hair, which is likely to be fragile. Hair Expert Helen Owens notes: "The hair goes through different stages during regrowth, and the degree of scalp discomfort varies from person to person. So I think it's best to work closely with a client's medical team and see first what the doctor and/or dermatologist recommends. She may prescribe a particular line of topical creams and/or regrowth products for the scalp, and/or may suggest a shampoo and/or conditioner that contains or is free of certain ingredients to help soften the follicle as it regrows."

Visit your hairdresser soon after your hair starts to regrow to create a plan of action to deal with the stages of regrowth. He or she can also help with sophisticated options for improving your looks. As crazy as it sounds, we recommend that you cut your hair as soon as it grows in about an inch. You may not want to part with even a tiny fraction of your new hair, but just nipping off the dead ends can really help the shape and improve the thickness. See tips on getting a great pixie cut in our FAQs section.

Color after Treatment

Most hair stylists encourage you to wait until your hair is a few inches long to color it. Even then, what kind of color makes a difference, and you should opt for something gentle, possibly semipermanent over permanent colors and bleach. Here are some tips from celebrity colorist Corey Powell:

- To cover gray or just add richness to your own color, try nonammonia, nonperoxide tints and stains. Some brands include Herbatint, which is natural. Clairol Touch is good as well. During this time, it is important to look as good as you can!
- For any color, try a low or nonammonia color like Redken Shades EQ, L'Oreal Dia-Light or Dia-Richesse, or Inoa. Avoid bleach, ammonia, or high levels of peroxide!
- If your hair has become really curly and uncontrollable, consider a keratin treatment. They are great at smoothing out wiry hair.

HAIR RESTORATION: TEMPORARY OPTIONS

Extensions.

If you want to have long hair again immediately, you might try extensions. Extensions can give a natural lush look when done properly. At the same time, improperly applied extensions can look false and can place a lot of stress on the scalp and hair, causing bald patches (called *traction alopecia*). Even if you are already done with chemotherapy, check in with your oncology team before trying any hair augmentation. Helen Owens elaborates: "Any good attachment should have the approval of the client's medical team. Chemotherapy is a serious treatment that dramatically affects the entire body, so we want to make sure whatever is worn on the head is medically congruent."

If your hair is two to three inches long, you can try extensions, especially if you're working with varying lengths of hair on the head (patchiness, hair that's longer in one area and shorter in another, etc.). Helen Owens notes: "Oftentimes I will combine several methods to get a finished look that's also comfortable for the client. What women need to remember is that with appropriate styling and design, they can achieve *any* look they want; the key is using the attachment method and correct application."

Toni Love adds: "Keratin-tipped extensions and fusion tend to be best for people who have short or medium hair. Interlocking (where there are no braids and glue) is another popular technique used to apply hair extensions for volume as well as length. The application time is much shorter, and the results are great!"

Hair Integration Systems.
Another method of nonsurgical hair replacement is hair integration systems such as the Intralace prosthesis created by Lucinda Ellery (available only in the UK, but there are versions in the United States too). A hair integration system serves as a wig and extensions in one and can be used with as little as an inch and a half of regrowth. A sheer mesh is placed over your head, through which any existing hair is pulled and braided. Hair wefts are then attached to the braids and blended in. It does not hide or inhibit new hair growth. Done correctly, they are virtually undetectable.

Linda explains: "This at first may act as a wig, but as soon as hair starts to regrow, this system will allow full integration with the new hair coming through without the need to cut or shave natural hair, an added plus when after treatment you want to retain whatever hair has grown in!" The effect is very natural and allows freedom to wash, swim, and otherwise treat hair as if it is your own. It costs about $1,500 to $3,000 and can last two years with regular touch-ups.

Hair Restoration: Permanent Surgical Hair Replacement

On rare occasions, hair does not regrow after cancer treatment. In this case there are several sophisticated surgical hair replacement techniques to consider.

NeoGraft or micrograft.
In this new hair replacement technique in which thousands of hair follicles are removed from thick areas of hair and implanted into thinning areas. It is

a minimally invasive procedure done in a dermatologist's office under light sedation. The results can be virtually undetectable—a far cry from the "hair plugs" of the past.

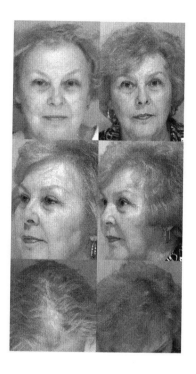

Hair Transplantation by Dr. James Marotta

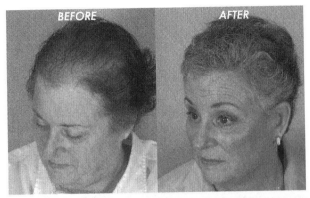

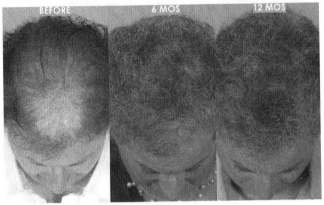

Micrograft hair transplant, by Dr. Alan J. Bauman

Low-light laser therapy (LLLT).

A noninvasive treatment using a noncutting laser beam to stimulate hair growth, approved by the FDA in 2007. Dr. Alan Bauman explains: "One theory of how this hair loss treatment works is that it stimulates the production of energy at the cellular level: therefore, improving cell function. European studies have shown that LLLT stops hair loss in 85 percent of cases and stimulates new hair growth in 55 percent of cases. While LLLT is no 'miracle cure' for hair loss, we have found similar results with our patients." At-home LLLT devices are also now available.

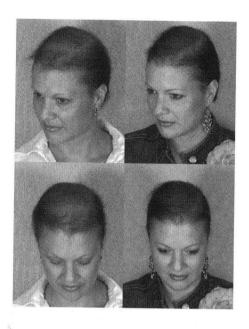

Laser Cap Treatment for chemotherapy patient: before
and 4 months after, by Dr. Alan J. Bauman

Supplements.

Dermatologists and hair replacement experts have found that some vitamin supplements can assist with thinning hair or hair regrowth. Two that seem promising are RegeneMax by Xymogen and Viviscal. Speak to your doctor.

Revivogen.

A new topical formulation made for female pattern baldness in particular. It is a promising new hair care system that works to block the production of DHT, the by-product of testosterone, which causes hair thinning and loss.

FREQUENTLY ASKED QUESTIONS

Will keeping my hair long before treatment starts make any hair thinning worse?
There is no evidence to suggest that long hair "weighs down" hair follicles or puts a strain on the roots. Some women opt to go short before treatment

to ease the pain of hair release or get ready for a wig fitting, but the choice to stay long is entirely yours.

Will wearing a wig stunt my hair regrowth?
The short answer is no, according to Linda Ellery. In fact, keeping your scalp warm and protected is the best way to encourage regrowth.

I'm worried about my kids' reaction to my hair loss.
One of the most visible characteristics of cancer treatment is lost or thinning hair, and you may feel it is important to prepare friends, family, and coworkers for any changes—particularly if you want to keep your treatment private. Even if you later opt for a wig that does not match your current style, a sudden style change can be surprising and sometimes alarming. It's probably best to have a frank discussion with adults who may be affected by the change in your appearance. Very small children, however, may need extra assurance that their mothers and other relatives are OK. Here are some ideas and stories:

- Consider having your hair cut in two stages: first shorter, and then go really short. This gives kids time to adjust to a new look so that the eventual change won't be so surprising.
- Barry Hendrickson suggests you go one step further with older kids and ask them to accompany you to the wig salon: "A grown daughter can be a great help with her sense of current fashion trends. This can become an excellent opportunity for sharing special time together."
- Let children touch the wig and try it on. This helps demystify it.
- Jodie Guerrero, author of *Jodie's Journey,* found that her children actually adapted easily: "The first time, my hair was shaved in hospital and my kids were really little. The second time, we made it a bit of an event at home with a hair-dresser, and they got bored with it pretty quick and ran off to play with their toys. We thought they would either cry from fright or laugh—but they did neither and it made no

difference. In fact, they carried on as if nothing had changed. This showed me that kids don't really care what Mummy/Daddy look like—they love you regardless."

Cancer strategist Elyn Jacobs shares these additional tips:

- Acknowledge fears—let them know you want to hear their fears and thoughts.
- Remain calm and in control—if you appear anxious or fearful, your children will emulate that fear.
- It's OK to appear sad—this will let them know it is safe to express their feelings.
- Make every attempt to keep your child's routine as stress-free and normal as possible. As hard as it may be, try to maintain extracurricular activities, playdates, and family fun.
- Employ art as a venue for your children to express their feelings. This helps children put their fears to paper and therefore externalize them. And a tangible item like a drawing or sculpture gives you a wonderful opportunity to discuss your illness with them in a different, less scary way.

Will extensions after cancer treatment slow my new hair regrowth?
No. Just be sure your hair is strong enough to bear the extensions, and opt for short ones over long, heavy ones.

Hair extensions can be costly. Any chance they can be covered by insurance as part of my healing?
The answer is maybe. Helen Owens comments: "A "cranial prosthesis" is a hair loss solution that can be covered by some insurance, and if a practitioner has the skill to combine methods and techniques, she can custom create/design a nonsurgical hair replacement solution that meets the insurance requirements. That may include using hair extensions as part of that solution."

I want to switch to natural hair products during treatment. What ingredients should I look for?

Toni Love: "Many women opt for natural hair products such as shea butter and olive oil to prevent dry and brittle hair. Both products add moisture to the hair shaft without leaving a 'greasy' film. Products containing rosemary extract have a rejuvenating effect, and the extract helps reduce headaches and swelling. Many women like natural shampoos that contain soap bark extract, which allows it to foam on the hair shaft."

I know natural hair requires a lot of styling, and I don't want a wig that needs the same.

Isaac Mann: "Go with a synthetic wig if you have difficulty styling your natural hair. It goes without saying: if it takes a lot to style your own hair, you will have the same trouble styling a human hair wig."

My scalp feels tender at night. Any suggestions?

Try a satin pillowcase like those made by Savvy Sleepers (www.savvysleepers.com). Or you can consider a sleep cap: these are very soft skullcaps that come in a variety of soothing fabrics, such as cotton interlock and fleece. They can buffer your scalp from irritation and keep you cooler, or warmer, depending on the fabric.

I have heard there is "virgin" and "descaled" human hair wigs. Can you explain?

Barry Hendrickson: "Virgin European hair still has its cuticle. It possesses a wonderful luster and color as well as its natural curl pattern…one of the softest [types of] hair. Descaled hair has the cuticle removed by a chemical process to keep it from tangling when washed. Descaled hair is straighter hair and often used to blend with other types of hair to produce a softer refined hair."

I have really long hair and hate to "waste" it by cutting it off. Is there anything I can do?

You can give back your "lost" hair to a foundation that provides wigs for women and children who can't afford them such as Locks of Love (www.

locksoflove.org) or Children with Hair Loss (www.childrenwithhairloss. us). Many organizations will take colored or permed hair too! Check individual websites for requirements about hair type and length.

I'm thinking about getting a "fun" wig. Any suggestions?
Some survivors choose to have fun with their wigs and even have several that range from natural to "out there," using them to reflect different sides of their personalities. The decision is entirely yours, but whichever you choose, approach wig wearing as a *choice* that empowers you to face each day with courage. Here are a few survivors' stories.

- I found a wig [very different from my usual hair] that was styled after Victorian Beckham's short blond haircut, and I was hooked. I got all my hair trimmed off and started wearing 'Victoria,' and it turned out to be so much fun... The compliments kept coming in. It seemed like every week someone stopped me to compliment me on my wig. 'Victoria' sure helped me get through my treatment with style!" — Nancy Stephans
- "I wish I had known how fun it was to get wigs...because like most people I dreaded shaving my head. But I got two wigs made and each had its own identity. One was long and matched my natural hair color...and a radical new look that I called the 'Gina Gershon' with... a luscious cocoa color. 'Gina' attracted a different attention...it was really fun to have two egos, two different personalities." —Jennifer Alhasa, cancer coach
- "I never did get the courage to go natural (maybe next time), but I ended up trading in the cap for a platinum blonde wig. I was trying on wigs at Lulu's (opened by a breast cancer survivor) and after trying out several sedate brunette/red wigs, I spotted a blonde bombshell wig up in the corner. (I'd never been a blonde!) It was bold and very different from any look I'd had before. It gave me a feeling that I had a choice in the midst of a situation I did not choose. It made me feel like myself – adventurous! My advice is this: think of this as an

opportunity to try something new. It's empowering. Have an adventure, whether you go natural or try something edgy, chic or just plain fun. Life is short - be bold!" - Monica Doyle, PhD

What is the best way to care for my scarves and head covering?
During cancer treatment, it is more important than ever to keep whatever fabrics that touch your skin extra clean.

It is OK to machine wash most cotton scarves (like bandanas), but hand washing is best to preserve the color and life of your piece. Here are step-by-step instructions courtesy of www.scarves.net:

- Fill a sink or large bowl with cool water.
- Add a small amount of mild detergent and make suds.
- Submerge your scarf fully in the water. Knead and squeeze it through the suds until it's totally wet.
- Let the scarf sit in the water for approximately fifteen minutes.
- Drain or pour out the water.
- Rinse your scarf by holding it under cool tap water. Squeeze and run it under the faucet until the water runs clear through the scarf and there are no suds left.
- Squeeze water out of your scarf—be gentle! Don't wring the fabric too hard.
- Lay your scarf on a towel and roll the towel; this step will eliminate a good amount of dampness so it can dry.
- Unroll the towel and lay your scarf on a dry towel to dry completely. Never hang a scarf to dry—doing this could damage its fibers!

When you hand wash silk scarves, add an extra step: after rinsing the scarf, refill your bowl or sink with cool water and add a tiny splash of distilled white vinegar. Swish the scarf around, and then rinse again. The vinegar helps the silk keep its sheen.

My everyday baseball hat has become boring. What are some other flattering styles?

Here are a few favorites:

- The slouchy hat (or slouchy beanie) is a soft cap with extra fabric at the crown that drapes behind the head. Slouchy hats come in a wide assortment of soft fabrics, including microfleece and cashmere and are very hip these days.
- The snood dates from the 1940s and is now widely worn by the rockabilly and retro crowd. Traditionally it is a close-fitting net hood that would cover a bun, but modern-day versions are often hand-crocheted and cover the head from the hairline, capturing any hair in it. They are soft and comfortable, and they offer full head protection.
- Floppy hats are wide-brimmed hats that usually come in straw or fabric, drape the face beautifully, and give excellent coverage with the bonus of generous sun protection. They can be endlessly customized by wrapping scarves and look great with oversize sunglasses.

I'd love to get a professional keratin treatment now that I have "chemo curls," but they are costly.

Keratin treatments are the gold standard for straightening hair, but they are come at a price—usually three hundred dollars and up. Celebrity Colorist Corey Powell recommends the Pravana Keratin Fusion Texture Control Kit, which is done at home. It is easy to use and costs less than fifty dollars. Corey recommends you get a friend to help with the back of your head for the most even results.

Can I add a bit of scent to my wig to freshen it up?

Lisa Lewis, creator of Wig It2: "Take a [cotton swab], dip it in vanilla extract, and gently wipe inside the wig cap or across the weft of hair extensions. Let air dry and enjoy a light, attractive vanilla smell to your hair."

My hair isn't growing in as fast as I would like. When can I start using extensions?
There is no length requirement for the natural hair to which extensions can
adhere. The key is finding a method that works for the hair you have. Helen
Owens reassures: "My creations can be done with no hair or as little as one inch
of hair. For hair this short a client would be a candidate for nonsurgical hair
replacement. Nonsurgical hair replacement uses human hair from outside the
client to create a prosthesis that is not surgically implanted, but can be attached
on a semipermanent basis and can be worn three to four months at a time."

How do I get the best pixie cut?
Corey Powell: "Face shape is important when considering cutting hair short:

- *Round face*: This means width of your forehead, cheekbones, and
  jaw are all equal, with soft features (like Charlize Theron). You want
  to create height and length, with a spiky top, short sides, and wispy
  neckline.
- *Square face*: Consider yourself lucky if you have a strong angular
  jawline like Demi Moore. If you need to play down the jawline, add
  lots of texture, especially around the edges. Spiky cuts and off center
  parts work great.
- *Heart-shaped face*: Your face is wider at the forehead and gently
  narrows down, sometimes with a bit of a pointy chin (think Reese
  Witherspoon). Draw attention to the eyes and cheekbones with a
  sweeping side bang to break up your forehead. You may want to balance the chin by showing some hair at the neckline or behind the ear.
- *Oval face*: Congrats, you have the most versatile face shape (like Ann
  Hathaway). To find your most flattering style, determine what are
  your best features (eyes, cheekbones, etc.) and highlight that with
  your haircut.
- While most hair textures will work with a pixie, curly hair can be difficult. Your hairdresser will need to cut deliberate chunks and use a
  Keratin treatment to smooth out a bit.

- To avoid a hard "razor" look, tell your hairdresser cut into your hair. This is called "slice cutting" and helps give a piece-y look.
- To give your pixie some definition, use a paste. My favorite right now is Shu Uemura Clay Definer Rough Molding Pomade.
- When it is time to grow out...Learn how to use clips and pins; make it fun. Go as long as you can in between cuts. And adding in some color always helps ease the transition too.

My wig has picked up some everyday smells. What can I do?
Lisa Lewis: "Use white vinegar to wipe out smoke, mildew, or sweaty odors in your hair or wigs. Simply mix one teaspoon of white vinegar and one pint of tap water. Pour into a spray bottle and mist hair/wig to quickly stop the odor. Let air dry or blow dry on cool."

HAIR TIPS FROM SURVIVORS

"Make sure to have your hair cut, colored, and washed before surgery, and don't skimp on going to a local salon to have your hair washed and dried afterward when mobility is a challenge. It feels so good to have someone scrub your head, especially when you can't lift your arms up to wash and style it." —Elizabeth Thompson, MD, cancer previvor and founder of BFFL Co.

"This is my second time of bald due to chemotherapy. As my hair was falling out this time, I decided to have fun with it. My first hairdo was a Skrillex [a long Mohawk]. Then I colored it cobalt blue. Next was a teal mohawk.

"By the time all of my hair was gone, the weather was still hot, so I went bald in public. I was an out-of-the-closet cancer patient and got a lot of stares from men. Several women told me that I looked beautiful. I guess I gave off a comfortable vibe because strangers started touching me. The first person held my hand. Then I got cornered by two women at a store who insisted on hugging me. Next someone came up to me in a waiting room and kissed me on the cheek. Whoa! Support is nice, but respect my boundaries, people!

"Being bald in public has taught me that wigs are for other people's comfort, not mine. I hope that all bald women can feel empowered to go hairless in public. Just beware of strangers. Maybe we should wear a button that reads, 'Yes, I have ovarian cancer. No, I don't want a hug. And please don't tell me about your friend who died from ovarian cancer.'" —Lynne Wendler

"I've found that the best wigs have dark roots so your parts look natural." —Lynn Jones

"I had a head shaving party the week before my hair was due to fall out. This made it on my terms. I was surrounded by loved ones, and we had fun doing it. My nine-year-old daughter got to shave my hair into a mohawk, which she loved and made it easier for her. When my buzzed hair fell out, it was less traumatic (and less mess)." -- Meagan Farrell, creator of Clear the Clutter Personal Organizing

"In order to help my young nieces and nephews not be afraid of what I was going through with my cancer, I let them try on my wigs whenever they wanted to. After my hair grew back they continued to ask me if my hair was a wig or my real hair." —Rebecca Cagle, professional life coach

"A must-have with a head scarf is a cotton padded hat liner to wear underneath it. It makes your bald head look fuller. They are made of 100 percent cotton terrycloth and can be purchased from TLC Cancer Care Catalog. Tying headscarves takes practice and patience: a good how-to book was written by a chemo patient. It is called *Tie One On* and is available at www.teal-books.com." —Jori Walker, three-year survivor

"My own personal feeling is that hair makes me feel like me and not a sick person. I hated being pitied or coddled or not treated like me anymore. When I wear my [natural-looking wig], I can go about my day with dignity." —Janet Crain

"How we each manage our survivorship is as unique as we are as individuals. I made a decision that I did not want to look like a cancer survivor because if I look healthy it helps me to feel healthy... I had my wig styled similarly to my usual style. People did not know I was wearing a wig. It was pretty amazing. I frequently would lift a corner of the wig to prove it." — Suzanne Flavin

"My hair growth was very slow after treatment. My hair grew back very thin and bald at the crown, as I found many women experienced. My dear friend who has lived every day for four years with stage 4 breast cancer suggested I visit her dermatologist who helped grow back her hair. Dr. Sumayah Taliaferro started me on cortisone scalp injections to stimulate and regrow my hair follicles, as well as prescribed minoxidil. Though my hair texture is not as thick as before treatment, my bald spot is disappearing." —Mya D.

"I developed a really nasty and very painful bout of folliculitis of my scalp when I lost my hair to the chemo. I didn't want any more drugs so I created a soothing scalp serum that resolved the infection in about a week...little did I know that this would be the start to my skincare line Botanicals for Hope! After resolving the infection on my scalp, I was very careful how I cleansed not only my head but everywhere else on my body since the chemo left me virtually hairless. No hot water, using a gentle, all-natural botanically enriched all-over body wash, dabbing not rubbing myself dry, and applying a lotion that would not clog pores or follicles." —Kimberly Luker, founder of Botanicals for Hope, www.botanicalsforhope.com

"Shave your head as soon as it starts to itch badly before it falls out. I did so and my hair never fell out; it just stayed looking like it was shaved. I walked around with a shaved head and got more compliments on my beautiful head than I ever did when I had hair!" —Audrey Darrow, president of Earth Source Organics

"When my hair started to fall out after my first treatment, my hair stylist gave me a cute, spiky cut. After the second treatment, when it really was falling out, she offered to shave my head in a private room. 'No,' I said. 'Do it here in the salon. I'm not afraid or ashamed. And someone here may have to go through it one day.'

"My strategy for dealing with the 'visible' part of my cancer treatment was simple: I looked at myself long and hard in the bathroom mirror at the start of each day. 'Cry,' I said, out loud. 'Get it out *now*, in the next five minutes, because that's all you get today.' Very quickly, cry turned into laugh. How *ridiculous*, I thought…*laugh*, yes, *that's* what I need to do!

"I wore a wig (hated it) to work, as I had just started a new job three weeks before my diagnosis. I put the thing on in the car when I got to work, and took it off as soon as I got back in the car to go home. I alternated between wigs and silky scarves. I hated those too. As soon as hair began to reasonably cover my head, I shed both wigs and scarves, at the encouragement of one of my African-American colleagues, who had close-shorn hair, by choice. She welcomed me to the 'sisterhood.' She gave me courage." —Annamarie DeCarlo

"My first wrestle with cancer, my hair only started to fall out when I started on a second round of stronger chemo called (R-CHOP). I woke up one morning and had a very sore scalp, so sore I could barely touch it. It was painful for two days, and then the pain went away, and then little by little all my hair started to come out, slowly at first.

"In hospital, I was shielded by the air conditioning and didn't feel the tropical heat on my head or the uncomfortable sweating that a wig caused in our subtropical weather in Queensland. I also did not want to wear a wig in the ward. Although, I did show it off to the hospital staff and gave a doctor the fright of his life when I tiptoed up behind him with this huge flowing wig—he jumped out of his skin when he saw me—all the nurses laughed at his reaction.

"To stop my wig from budging, I simply wore it further down on my head and stretched it a bit to fit over my scalp. If you choose the wrong wig and it is not fitted properly, it will fall off. Cancer patients wanting a good wig should make sure they choose the correct size or have someone check it for them. If it is the right size, it should not need 'sticking.'

"I never spent much on my wigs, and I would encourage women to not be too concerned about what the wig is made of (either synthetic or human hair)—the cost of human hair is far too great for most cancer patients, and to be honest, few people will notice the difference.

"I did not 'care' for my scalp with lotions and potions. I simply kept it warm and protected and made sure I was careful with the sun. Our tropical climate means the sun is extremely strong here, and you must make sure a bald head is covered with sunscreen and protected. I pretty much avoided the sun altogether. On formal occasions, I twisted turbans around my head to create pretty colors and beautiful designs.

"The main product I have always used is Dove everything. I didn't need to wash my hair (rarely)—as during my treatments it was a like 'baby fluff.' However, I did wash my head most times when I had a shower, just to feel clean, and used my regular Dove body wash on my head. No need to really use shampoo and conditioner—until it started to grow back." —Jodie Guerrero, author of *Jodie's Journey*

"I've always had pretty long hair, and I began losing my hair within one week after my first treatment. So I had my stylist cut my hair short. Within a few weeks I looked like the 'fuzzy' weeds in the yard! I wore wigs during this time, which was a chore for me. I washed my head often and used olive oil as a moisturizer. After my fifth treatment (I had a total of six), my hair started to grow back really slowly. Now I can see more hair growth. I also sometimes use Sulfur8, which doesn't smell so good, but is proven to grow hair. I am looking forward to getting rid of the wigs and continuing to live my new normal!" —Jamila Davis

"I never wore wigs because cancer made me not feel like myself. So I went around bald or I wore fashionable hats that covered my whole head when I went out. When I went into the more severe chemo, I lost all the hair on my body. However, I started putting makeup on my eyes to make them pop, which I had never done as much. Then I found my new best friend, earrings. Long, dangly earrings. I began to appreciate having no hair.

"As my hair started growing back, I started loving a pixie cut. Cancer turned this consistently long-haired girl into a sassy pixie-cut gal. I am growing it out now because I want to donate to Locks of Love. I plan to cut it off again. The experience of having no hair was so freeing and taught me to see myself a different way. It taught me that 'It's only hair' really has a lot more truth to it than I ever thought. It gave me a new perspective on my ability to have short hair that I would never have learned otherwise." —Amber Lockwood

"I wore wigs for going out, but I wasn't comfortable. I wore cute hats and enjoyed the attention of other survivors coming up to me to offer me encouragement. Fight the cancer, but don't fight the encouragement of others." — Christine Peglar

"Here are my do's and don'ts for women who are going to undergo chemo and really want to wear a wig during hair loss:

1. Find a reputable wig salon. Check with your doctor, staff, chemo nurse, support group, the Internet. A good salon will have a staff with the training to help you select the style, color, and length for you. They will have the ability to cut hair as well.

2. Visit the wig salon before you go into chemo. It will help the beautician to be able to see your current hair color, texture, style. A good salon will have many choices for you.

3. Relax. This is an opportunity for you to try out all the hair colors and styles you secretly wondered, 'How would I look with red hair or a curlier style?' You will have a pro to help you.

4. Have the hairpiece trimmed to your face. A good wig salon will be able to professionally trim your hair to your liking, and learn the proper way to put the wig on. This is very important to making your hair look natural, your own and not 'wiggy.'

5. It is best to use less brushing and more 'hand fluffing,' as the wigs I like are prestyled. Usually a little shake of the head and a little pushing it into place with your hands works well.

6. Buy the best quality you can afford. If this is out of the question financially, check support groups and Look Good, Feel Better, as they may have slightly used wigs to donate.

7. Don't let the well-meaning family and friends unduly influence you with well-meaning comments. Even support groups and survivors cannot really know how you feel about your appearance and sense of wellbeing. Others may not mind wearing a scarf or a hat or even just going bare-headed. If that isn't you, don't let others make you feel you are not strong or that you are hiding something by wanting to wear a wig.

Finally, allow yourself time to mourn your loss of hair. Hair is a big thing! Once you have allowed for the pity party, put on your wig. Wow, you look so good!" —Mary Fedor

"Here's the story about my wig. When I went shopping for a wig it was difficult. I wasn't feeling well, and my hair was falling out. But then I found a wig that was styled after Victorian Beckham's short blond haircut, and I was hooked....The compliments kept coming in. All I had to do was pop her on in the morning, and my hair looked great. It never got frizzy or flat.

"Dealing with wind was pretty funny though. It would blow straight out and stay there. My husband and I had more laughs about the wig. Sometimes it would ride up on my head, and he would touch his forehead to signal that it needed to be pulled down. One night I was having friends over for dinner and left my wig on the counter when I was cooking. When I went to put it back on I noticed that part of the bangs were melted. The steam from the dishwasher had damaged my wig, so I gave her a little haircut and popped it back on before my friends came!"—Nancy Stephans

"I decided during cancer treatment to stop coloring my hair. I figured my body was getting enough chemicals. I decided before radiation to ditch shampoos with a lot of chemicals, parabens, etc. I pamper my hair with good, more organic shampoos. I only used semipermanent hair color. My hair is now graying and whitening slowly and naturally, and it is OK." —Carla Joy Zambelli, www.ihavebreastcancerblog.me

"I had a head-shaving party to help me deal with the loss. I figured having a party was the best way to prepare myself. We cut my hair super short and then tried to get it into a Mohawk, but none of us were skilled, so we teased the heck out of it and spray-painted it pink. I then tried on a bunch of hats and silly wigs to the enjoyment of all of my girlfriends. We made pink drinks (pink lemonade and vodka), had a bunch of appetizers, and giggled all afternoon. It was a truly special occasion, and it made losing my hair bearable." —Christine Peglar

"I did not like wigs: too itchy. I wore baseball caps. I felt like being obviously bald explained to people around me why I was slower or using the electric carts. I think people were nicer and more patient as a result." —Meagan Farrell, Clear the Clutter Personal Organizing

"I found wigs extremely itchy and uncomfortable and almost always wore a hat. I ended up wedded to a knit hat with a microfleece lining that was very comfortable and warm, but ugly. One wonderful person made me a couple of really cute knit hats, which I also wore.

"I would suggest that you look for at least four or five head-covering options. Check them for itchiness if possible against tender skin like your stomach. If you are getting treatment in the winter, think about warmth. We lose a lot of body heat from the head and even more so when you have no hair." —Rebecca Bogart, author of "From Chemo to Carnegie Hall," www.rebeccabogart.com

"I regularly gave my Mum Indian head massages when she lost her hair through chemo. This stimulates the blood flow to the hair follicle and encourages nice, thick regrowth. Needless to say her hair returned as beautiful as it was before the treatment." —Cindy Woodward, skin-care therapist at the Beauty Retreat Organic Day Spa, Sheffield, England

"If you don't like wearing a wig, then don't. Take it off, throw it up in the air, put it on your dog. Whatever you want. If you love it, keep it. It will be a nice change of pace once your hair grows back." —Angelique Neumann, founder of RN Cancer Guides, www.rncancerguides.com

"The best tip I received for tying head scarves securely is to use a wide rubber-coated hair band or scrunchie in a color that matches your scarf to anchor it. Also be sure to purchase scarves that are made of lightweight cotton or other woven fabric so they don't slip off your head. Silk scarves do not work as well, but they are great to add color over the top of another scarf as a 'finisher scarf.' A thirty-six-inch square or a very long oblong scarf works the best." —Jori Walker, three-year survivor

"I made a homemade conditioner out of water, apple cider vinegar, honey, and a dab of coconut oil—I love that! I just read about using cinnamon, honey, and olive oil—put it on your head where the hair is thin for thirty minutes and then wash it off—so I'm excited to try that." —Wendy Kuhn

"I am one of the 6 percent that *permanently* lost their hair due to Taxotere, a chemo poison that saved my life. There is a lot to be said about hair loss and the emotional side. You have to wrap your head and heart around what you really are as a person rather than your outward identity. At first, I tried to use the time to experiment with different hair colors and styles, but I quickly learned that it would not work for me. I looked like different people. My job is in marketing, and part of the goal in marketing is to be memorable. I now have a wig that is my style, and I know the difference between a good wig and a bad one. The best advice I can give is get one that has darker roots and highlights. No one even knows I wear a wig now, and I have been asked where I get my hair done. It's hilarious." —Lynn Jones

"Wigs: have fun with them, and try to stay away from ones with too much shine. Make your wig your own by having it custom cut and by accessorizing it. Remember, the color and cut isn't permanent. Also wig tape should be your new best friend. It also prevents the silky head wraps from falling off. Try to buy wraps with patterns and again, accessorize the look. Earrings, clip-on flowers, and fabulous makeup will distract everyone, even yourself at times." —Marlena Ortiz, young cancer survivor and founder of beating-cancerinheels.org

CHAPTER THREE

BREAST RECONSTRUCTION

IF YOU HAVE HEARD THE WORDS "I am sorry, but the tumor in your breast is cancerous," you know what stomach-turning, nauseating fear feels like. Survival and recovery are primary concerns, but what your breast(s) will look like and how long the reconstruction process will take is also up there. All of a sudden you are faced with making decisions about types of surgery such as lumpectomy vs. mastectomy. Which is better? If mastectomy, what kind? How does reconstruction work? And what, most importantly, what can you expect as a final result? You have to make choices about things that you know very little, choices that will affect you for the rest of your life. All the while, terrifying images flash in your head.

People say that when it comes to cancer, the treatment may be more devastating than the diagnosis. Invasive surgery is more often than not part of breast cancer treatment. Even in this day and age, some women opt out of lifesaving surgeries because of the fear of losing a breast. A breast for a woman is part of her femininity, and a loss of one or both breasts can be a big blow to self-esteem. It does not help that the Internet is full of images of huge scars against flat chests and that some doctors do not refer to a reconstructed breast as breast tissue…or even offer reconstruction.

We are here to tell you that with patience and proper decision making, you can emerge from a terrible experience being very happy with the results and looking beautiful. No woman asks for breast cancer. You may have never thought of plastic surgery as something you would do. Yet, it does not mean that you should not take advantage of sophisticated, modern developments in the fields of reconstruction and plastic surgery. Many talented, dedicated medical professionals have worked to develop techniques and skills to create wonderful aesthetic results with little, if any, scarring and natural looking reconstructed breast. This is *not* "your mother's mastectomy."

This chapter will break it all down and empower you with knowledge to make the right choice for yourself. We will discuss the pros and cons of many reconstructive procedures, talk about what to look for in a plastic surgeon, and show you images of beautifully reconstructed breasts. We will explain that you can proceed with reconstruction right away or wait to do it when you are ready. Also, we will warn you about anything that can hinder good results. You will understand the time span of your recovery so that you can properly manage your expectations.

You should keep several things in mind to achieve success.

1. Choose a Board-Certified Plastic Surgeon

Involve a board-certified plastic surgeon in your decision about breast surgery—whether you opt for reconstruction or not. A plastic surgeon will work with your oncologic surgeon to determine the best placement of incisions and make recommendations about reconstruction based on your type of cancer, body type, health, and desired outcome. Even if you do not plan to reconstruct now, you may wish to do so in the future.

2. Assemble a Team and Coordinate the Process

Make your reconstruction part of your healing process. Make your plastic surgeon part of your oncology team. The timing of your reconstruction must be coordinated with your radiation or chemotherapy treatments. Let your oncologist know that you are in the process of reconstruction. For example, for the most part, surgery cannot be performed while you are going through chemotherapy. If you are not planning a one-step reconstruction, then you may want skin expanders (discussed later in the chapter) to already be in place prior to starting chemo treatments. Certain reconstruction procedures cannot be done on irradiated skin. Understanding your options will be crucial.

3. Educate Yourself and Plan Carefully

Take time to ask questions and read this chapter carefully. It takes a while for cancer to develop in the body—actually years. Unless you are told differently by your doctor (and depending on the staging of your cancer), *you have time* to find the right plastic surgeon, see pictures and examples of his or her work, and speak to previous patients. With proper planning, you can avoid mistakes.

4. Be Patient

Understand that healing is a process, and getting the right results takes time and patience. Even if you have immediate reconstruction, it will not be one step. But do remember that there will be an end to your cancer treatment, and even if your only care right now is "getting cancer out of your body" today, a successful reconstruction of your breast will help your self-image and confidence forever.

5. Learn about Financial Options

Do not assume that you cannot afford reconstructive surgery. Insurance companies *must* cover reconstruction as part of your breast cancer treatment under law. Even if you do not have insurance, you do have options.

This chapter will explain:

- the path from diagnosis to surgery: managing expectations and costs
- choosing a plastic surgeon
- lumpectomy
- mastectomy
- reconstruction with implants
- reconstruction with tissue (flap reconstruction)
- nipple reconstruction and nipple tattooing
- FAQs
- checklist of questions for your doctor

Making decisions about what surgery to have can be overwhelming. However, this may be one of the most important steps you will ever take. Learning about options is the best way to be in control about your health and cosmetic outcome. As you will see from the pictures in this chapter, reconstructing the breast in its entirety, including a nipple and an areola, is now possible. It is also possible to customize the result for every woman. And it is possible to have a beautiful, natural result.

FROM DIAGNOSIS TO SURGERY

The period of time between diagnosis of cancer and surgery is often the most difficult time. You may be urged to make your choice about breast surgery quickly. You may feel an internal pressure to "have it done and over with," but you also need to take your time to make decisions. Few cancers will progress so quickly that waiting a week or two will truly matter. Surgical outcomes will affect you for the rest of your life.

You will meet with a breast surgeon (oncologic surgeon) almost immediately after diagnosis. *We advise you to involve a plastic surgeon immediately* even though you may not want to have yet another consultation. A plastic surgeon can explain aesthetic outcomes of procedures and alleviate some of the stress about your appearance after surgery.

Managing Expectations

Modern reconstruction techniques yield beautiful results; however your breasts may look or feel different in the future. But not all change is bad. Lana Koifman puts it candidly: "If you can embrace this opportunity as a platform to be able to improve yourself, this is sort of your chance not to necessarily become a "Barbie doll," but to have improvements made to the things you didn't like about your breasts."

> *"When first diagnosed with cancer, the most natural and correct desire is to survive. However, do remember now that you may care how a scar looks in the future. Consulting and involving a plastic surgeon from the very beginning of any surgery can save pain and cost in the future."*
> —Lana Koifman

Managing Anxiety about the Cost of Breast Reconstruction

You may initially reject the idea of breast reconstruction because of the cost, but try to put this fear aside. Breast cancer is a medical diagnosis, not elective plastic surgery. The Women's Health and Cancer Rights Act (WHCRA) requires coverage for breast cancer surgeries following mastectomies. It was signed into law on October 1, 1998, and requires most group insurance plans and HMOs, including Medicare and Obamacare, that cover mastectomies to *also* cover breast reconstruction—whether it is done immediately or in the future. For more information on your legal rights to reconstruction, visit the US Department of Labor's website: www.dol.gov/ebsa/Publications/whcra.html.

> **DON'T IMMEDIATELY REJECT THE IDEA OF PLASTIC SURGERY.**
> *Plastic surgeon Dr. Danielle Deluca-Pytell explains: "There are patients who come into my office that are very frank and say, 'I would not have walked into a plastic surgery office before this diagnosis.' But it is very possible to make changes that will keep you looking your best...There's nothing vain about wanting to make your breast look like a breast. You don't have to expect that breast cancer is going to leave you deformed. There should be a lot of hope, because you can make a lot of changes."*

Something else to consider might be cancer insurance. Because so many people are now touched by the disease, many insurance companies make supplemental insurance available specifically for a cancer diagnosis. In addition to helping with co-pays, some insurance companies may offer cash advances for out-of-pocket expenses, including things you may not have thought of, such as travel expenses related to your treatment, specialists, childcare, car payments, and more. Check with your insurance company for more information.

Choosing a Plastic Surgeon

The medical and aesthetic outcomes from a lumpectomy or mastectomy lie in the hands of your surgeons. Because a lumpectomy is not considered plastic surgery, a surgical oncologist may perform it, and you may need to insist a plastic surgeon is involved. Please do so! Mastectomies with reconstruction, during surgery or down the road, will be done by both a breast surgeon and plastic surgeon, so both should be involved from the start. Here are some tips on how to choose your plastic surgeon:

- Ask the doctor who diagnosed you with cancer for recommendations, and see if you can interview former patients about their experiences.
- Ask other breast cancer survivors for referrals.
- Ask the surgeon if he or she specializes in reconstruction and what are his or her preferred techniques.
- Check out the surgeon's education, experience, and malpractice records. Ideally, your surgeon should be a member in good standing of the American Society of Clinical Oncology (ASCO). You can check at www.asco.org.
- Confirm that the surgeons you are considering are board-certified. This means they have participated in a residency program in both general and plastic surgery and have received specialized medical training. Board-certified surgeons have also passed a comprehensive oral and written exam. Plastic surgeons who have been board-certified must become re-certified every ten years and must participate in additional medical education to do so. The American Board of Medical Specialties (ABMS) publishes the official ABMS Directory of Board-Certified Medical Specialists (www.abms.org).
- Ask if the surgeon has training in the latest techniques.
- Investigate the surgeon's admitting hospital. Is it convenient to your home? Your work? Do you feel comfortable there? What is its reputation?
- Interview a surgeon thoroughly. You must feel that he or she has a high level of competency, experience, and understanding of your medical *and* aesthetic needs and concerns. A checklist of suggested questions appears at the end of the chapter.
- Ask if the surgeon participates in clinical trials: this can sometimes mean that he or she is aware of and open to new and innovative techniques.

- Ask to see before-and-after images. Ask for both the best and worst results your surgeon had. It's important to be realistic!
- Finally: trust your gut. A good emotional connection is a must.

TYPES OF BREAST SURGERY: LUMPECTOMY AND MASTECTOMY

There are generally two types of breast surgery: lumpectomy and mastectomy. You will work with your medical team to make a decision about which is best in treating your cancer. Both procedures have their pros and cons from an aesthetic standpoint, which we detail below.

Lumpectomy (Breast-Conserving Surgery)

A lumpectomy is a procedure in which a cancerous tumor is surgically removed from the breast, along with a thin rim of tissue around the tumor to insure that all cancerous cells have been removed.

A lumpectomy removes *only* the lump, and it therefore saves much of the breast. A lumpectomy is usually followed by daily radiation for five to seven weeks to kill off any cancerous cells that may remain.

About 50 percent of women diagnosed with breast cancer are appropriate candidates for lumpectomy: this can be great news if you wish to keep much of your natural breasts, the same sensation in the affected breast, and, in some cases, the same appearance after your surgery.

The success of a lumpectomy from a cosmetic standpoint relies on two things: size of the breasts or tumor/breast ratio and type and location of tumor. The aesthetic results will typically be better if a woman has ample breasts or ones that she considers too large and wishes to have smaller, lifted breasts. Dr. Danielle Deluca-Pytell explains: "[Lumpectomy] can be combined with a medical reconstructive procedure such as a breast lift or breast reduction which camouflages a lumpectomy defect, and rearranges the breast tissue in a way that is cosmetically pleasing by lifting the nipple and removing excess skin."

Lumpectomy is generally more successful if the tumor is in a favorable location, usually in the inner or outer regions of the breast. If it is too close to the nipple or involves the nipple, it will not yield good aesthetic results.

It may initially seem that saving as much breast tissue of possible is attractive, but depending on the size of the tumor or if a patient has already had radiation, it may have devastating effects: "Changes can occur that are very difficult to undo and may involve having to do much more extensive surgery like tissue reconstruction from other parts of the body...sometimes more than once or sometimes involving a much larger part of the breast than expected, and then followed up by radiation," says Dr. Deluca-Pytell.

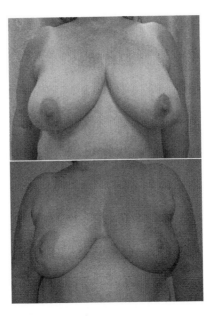

Lumpectomy reconstruction: Immediate left breast reconstruction after lumpectomy with breast reduction pattern, right breast reduction for symmetry, one year following completion of radiation therapy, by Dr. Danielle DeLuca-Pytell

Who Is a Good Candidate for Lumpectomy?

- You have a small, localized tumor: the most "ideal" areas are in the upper and outer quadrant of the breast because symmetry will not be affected as much by removal. A lumpectomy is not usually appropriate for multiple tumors.
- You have stage I or II breast cancer.

- You have no presence of inflammatory breast cancer (IBC) or extensive DCIS (ductal carcinoma in situ, abnormal or cancerous cells in milk duct of breast).
- You are willing to have radiation treatment afterward.
- Your breasts are large enough to sustain some tissue removal without distortion or poor aesthetic outcome, or you're interested in a breast reduction and tissue rearrangement at the same time.
- You have a pre-surgery diagnosis of cancer, and your surgeon knows where the cancer is. This way, your surgeon can use smaller incisions and rearrange the breast tissue around the site of surgery for better cosmetic results.
- You want to preserve normal nipple and skin sensation.
- Your cancer is not right next to or does not involve the nipple. In the case of nipple involvement, a more complicated procedure is necessary and the aesthetic outcome is not as predictable. That situation requires the removal of the nipple and areola as part of the lumpectomy, with reconstruction taking place later on.
- You want a procedure with as little downtime as possible.

Who Is Not a Good Candidate for Lumpectomy?
- You had a previous lumpectomy that did not remove all the cancer.
- You have cancer in two or more areas, IBC, or extensive DCIS.
- Your tumor is more than 5cm (2 inches) in diameter and cannot be shrunk by neoadjuvant chemotherapy prior to surgery.
- You have a known BRCA mutation and high risk for a second cancer.
- You are pregnant (follow-up radiation can harm an unborn child).
- You have very small breasts and a large tumor. A lumpectomy can sometimes create a dent or skin shrinkage in the breast. Maintaining or recreating symmetry may be difficult.
- Your tumor is located in the lower or inner part of the breast or near the nipple, which can increase chances of poor aesthetic outcome or even removal of nipple.

- You have had radiation in the past.
- You have a history of scleroderma (hardening of tissues), lupus (chronic inflammatory disease), or Hodgkin's disease (cancer of the lymphatic system).
- There are suspicious areas of breast calcification (which may be a sign of precancerous cells).
- Your schedule doesn't permit the intensive radiation schedule following surgery, you're sensitive to radiation, or you have a strong fear of radiation.
- You have a strong fear that your cancer will reoccur.
- You are unsure whether you will achieve the symmetrical outcome that a mastectomy plus reconstruction might be more likely to give.

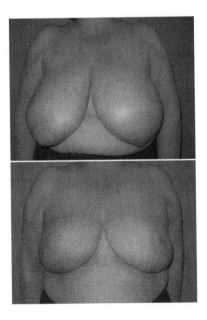

Lumpectomy reconstruction: Immediate right breast reconstruction after lumpectomy with breast reduction pattern, left breast reduction for symmetry, one year following completion of radiation therapy, by Dr. Danielle DeLuca-Pytell

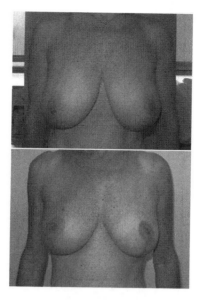

Lumpectomy reconstruction: Immediate right breast reconstruction after lumpectomy with breast reduction pattern, left breast reduction for symmetry, one year following completion of radiation therapy, by Dr. Danielle DeLuca-Pytell

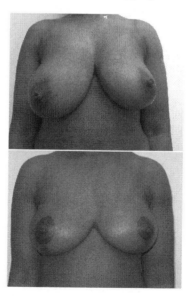

Lumpectomy reconstruction: Immediate left breast reconstruction after lumpectomy with breast reduction pattern, right breast reduction for symmetry, one year following completion of radiation therapy, by Dr. Danielle DeLuca-Pytell

Aesthetic Pros and Cons of Lumpectomy

Pros

- Maintain nipple and skin sensation, and your breast may look and feel the same as before surgery
- Less downtime than mastectomy usually requires
- You may not require reconstruction if it is done in conjunction with oncoplastic surgery

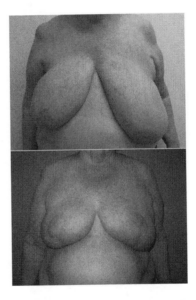

Lumpectomy reconstruction: Right breast reduction after prior lumpectomy and radiation, immediate left breast reconstruction utilizing breast reduction pattern after lumpectomy, by Dr. Danielle DeLuca-Pytell

Cons

- You may have poor aesthetic or medical outcome (skin puckering, dimples, asymmetry, loss of volume)
- Follow-up radiation may cause irreversible progressive breast shrinkage, asymmetry, deformity to the irradiated breast, scars, changes in skin color, spider veins, atrophy (wasting/shrinkage of tissue)
- Lumpectomy may cause lymphedema (swelling to the arm due to lymph node removal)

- You may have lingering pain
- Your breast may have delayed wound healing and be prone to infection

Mastectomy

A mastectomy is the surgical removal of the entire tissue of the breast under the skin. There are three basic types of mastectomy:

- Simple mastectomy. This procedure removes breast tissue, skin, and areola and nipple, but not the underarm lymph nodes. It can be used for noninvasive cancers such as DCIS or prophylactically to prevent breast cancer in women with BRCA or generally high risk. No axillary lymph nodes are taken, and recovery without is usually one to two weeks. This is the most common form of mastectomy performed today.
- Modified radical mastectomy. This procedure removes breast tissue, skin, areola and nipple, and some of the lymph nodes. It does not remove chest wall muscles. Recovery without reconstruction is usually two to three weeks.
- Radical mastectomy. Very rarely used these days, a radical mastectomy removes breast tissue, skin, areola and nipple, some chest wall muscles, and lymph nodes. It is used only with extensive cancer that has spread to the chest wall.

A mastectomy may not be necessary depending on your type of cancer. However, for most women, mastectomy with reconstruction has a better cosmetic outcome than does lumpectomy. From a medical standpoint, mastectomy usually does not require follow-up radiation.

Even if you don't even want to consider reconstruction after a mastectomy at this point, remember to let your surgeon know you may want reconstruction in the future so that he or she leaves enough skin and intelligent placement of incisions to yield the best aesthetic outcome.

Who Is a Good Candidate for Mastectomy?

- Cancer is found in multiple areas of your breast
- The tumor is more than 5cm (2 inches) in diameter and cannot be shrunk by neoadjuvant therapy prior to surgery
- You have a large tumor in a small breast
- A large area of tissue needs to be removed or the nipple and areola are involved
- Your breast has multiple calcifications
- You have a known BRCA mutation and high risk for recurrence
- Breast size and/or shape will not respond well to lumpectomy, or your cancer is in an area difficult to reach
- You have had a prior lumpectomy with radiation that did not remove all the cancer
- You have a history of scleroderma (hardening of tissues), lupus (chronic inflammatory disease), or Hodgkin's disease (cancer of the lymphatic system) that precludes radiation
- You don't want to have radiation.
- Your femininity and sexual self-image is not closely tied to having natural breasts
- The reduction or loss of natural sensation will probably not upset you
- You feel anxious that the cancer will return and want peace of mind

Who Is Not a Good Candidate for Mastectomy?

- Retaining your natural breasts is very important to you
- You wish to have a less complex surgery and a shorter recovery time
- You feel that lumpectomy alone will yield a good outcome

NEW MASTECTOMY TECHNIQUES

Several new mastectomy procedures aim to preserve as much breast tissue as possible for later reconstruction, at the same time as they reducing scarring. Reassure yourself that many sophisticated mastectomies today are not the crude, disfiguring ones of the past and can indeed be virtually scarless.

Skin-Sparing Mastectomy (SSM, or Subcutaneous Mastectomy)

In this technique, the surgeon removes breast tissue through a circular or elliptical incision around the areola and nipple. Although the areola and nipple are removed, the outer skin of the breast is left intact. The surgeon will then hollow out the breasts and perform a reconstruction with implants immediately, or put in an expander as a space holder for future reconstruction. The incision hole is closed with "purse-string sutures," which will be covered by later nipple reconstruction and tattooing, if desired.

An innovative variation on the skin-sparing mastectomy is called the "Box to X." In this technique, the incision is literally made in the shape of a box and the corners brought together when sutured shut. A box-shaped incision has two benefits: it gives the breast surgeon more than 25 percent more access for removing breast tissue, and allows the plastic surgeon to close the incision in two small lines. The scar is in the central portion of the breast and preserves some of the rounder shape of the breast. It can be virtually scarless, according to a recent article in *Annals of Plastic Surgery*.

Nipple-Sparing Mastectomy (NSM)

In this relatively new technique, the breast surgeon will make an incision around the nipple or around the outer breast and hollow out the breast, leaving the nipple and intact. The surgeon removes a bit of tissue beneath the nipple to be tested for cancerous cells and if they appear, the nipple will be removed and reconstructed later. If no cancer is detected, the breast will then be simultaneously reconstructed. The technique has the advantage of eliminating the need for future nipple reconstruction and leaves very little scarring.

Nipple-sparing mastectomy is usually appropriate for women with early stage breast cancer that is at least 2 centimeters away from the nipple area. It is also good for women with smaller breasts and small tumors or those doing a prophylactic mastectomy. The breast is usually reconstructed immediately, but in some cases an expander will be put in for future reconstruction. Women report positive results with this surgery.

At the time of this book, nipple-sparing mastectomy is increasingly considered as an alternative to skin-sparing mastectomy with higher rates of patient satisfaction and better self-image after surgery. However, because blood flow to the nipple is decreased after surgery, nipple hardening or deformation may result. Nerves to the nipple may be cut and sensation lost, as well.

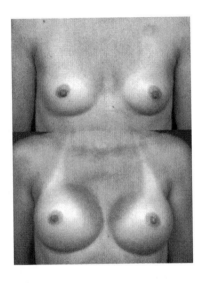

41 year old female following bilateral nipple sparing mastectomy with tissue expander, AlloDerm and injection of Botox into the pectoralis major muscle. Reconstruction completed with subsequent placement of Natrelle Style 20 round silicone implants and fat injection. By Dr. Allen Gabriel

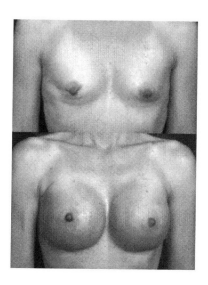

45 year old female following bilateral nipple sparing mastectomy with immediate reconstruction with tissue expander, AlloDerm and injection of Botox into the pectoralis major muscle. Reconstruction completed with placement of Natrelle Style 45 round silicone implants and fat injection. By Dr. Allen Gabriel.

Nipple and Areola-Sparing Mastectomy ("Keyhole" Mastectomy)

In nipple and areola-sparing surgery, the surgeon will make an incision around the side of the breast or the areola and hollow out the breast, leaving both the nipple and areola intact. This is a newer procedure that allows for the maximum preservation of tissue. Immediate reconstruction is usually performed, although in some cases an expander may be put in (see below).

As with NSM, because blood flow to the nipple is decreased after surgery, nipple hardening or deformation may result. This can require an additional surgery to correct. Nerves to the nipple are cut, so sensation can be lost as well.

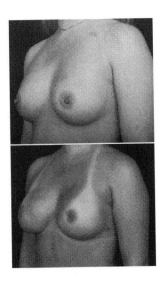

35 year old female following right nipple sparing and left areolar sparing mastectomy with immediate reconstruction with tissue expander, AlloDerm and injection of Botox into the pectoralis major muscle. Reconstruction completed with placement of Natrelle Style 45 round silicone implants. By Dr. Allen

Scar-Sparing Mastectomy

This procedure is very similar to the nipple- and areola-sparing mastectomy and aims at minimal scarring. The surgeon removes only the skin of the nipple, areola, and over the tumor. The breast tissue through the small incision—sometimes as little as two inches. Reconstruction can then be done with either implants or flap reconstruction transfer (see below). The benefit of this surgery is that it makes it easier to match the reconstructed breast with the unaffected breast. This surgery is appropriate for less invasive cancers.

BREAST RECONSTRUCTION

There are two techniques for breast reconstruction: breast implants or flap reconstruction, in which a new breast is formed from tissue taken from another part of the body. There are now many different kinds of tissue transfer that yield excellent cosmetic results. However, the American Society of Plastic Surgeons reported that the majority of women who had reconstruction chose implants and were happier with the outcome.

Prior to your mastectomy, speak with your surgeon about which method is best for you. If you have a unilateral mastectomy, you may wish to match your existing breast. If you have a bilateral mastectomy, you can choose the size and look of your new breasts. It is easier to achieve perfect symmetry when reconstructing both breasts, and many women now are opting for bilateral mastectomy for both prophylactic purposes and aesthetic outcomes. The choice is up to you.

Reconstruction with Breast Implants

Reconstruction with implants can be performed immediately (at the time of mastectomy) or later through the use of a tissue expander. Before any implant or expander is put in, the surgeon will create a pocket to hold it—usually the mastectomy incision to avoid additional resulting scars. Implants are placed under the layer of muscle within the breast because very little breast tissue is left from the mastectomy. Implants may require periodic MRI screening, and all types of implants affect mammogram readings. They may also need replacement down the line.

Implants are either saline or silicone, and the choice is personal. Insurance coverage is the same for either type of implant, so your surgeon should not have a financial motivation to choose one over the other.

Saline implants

Saline implants are comprised of an outer silicone shell filled with sterile salt water. They are inserted while empty and filled by the surgeon once in place.

Pros

- Firmer than silicone and offer more fullness (if you desire it)
- Easy to detect a rupture in a saline implant because it deflates. The saline leaking into the body is just absorbed without much health risk.

Cons

Can look hard and less natural.

Silicone Implants

Silicone implants come prefilled with silicone gel that closely mimics the feel of natural breast tissue. They were once banned, but are widely used today because they tend to look and feel more natural than saline. A recent study from the journal *Cancer* polled patients about their experience with implant reconstructive surgery: the women who opted for silicone implants were more satisfied with the look and feel of their breasts.

High-strength silicone gel implants ("gummy bear" implants) are becoming popular today and were approved by the FDA in February 2013. This type of gel is more stable and less apt to wrinkle or dimple than are some others. It may also yield a more natural teardrop-shaped contour. Like the candy for which they are nicknamed, "gummy bear" implants retain their shape after squished. These implants may have a lower rupture rate too.

Pros
- Softer and thought to be more natural than saline implants.

Cons
- More difficult to detect a rupture and more complicated surgery required to replace it due to leaking silicone into the body.

Who Is a Good Candidate for Reconstruction with Implants?
- You want to minimize scarring. Implants leave minimal scars to your breast only, whereas flap reconstruction leaves scars also at the sites that tissue is harvested.
- You are not pregnant and/or do not plan to breastfeed in the future.
- You want two shorter, simpler surgeries and less downtime
- You are willing to lose or alter your nonaffected breast to achieve symmetry
- You are not a smoker or are willing to quit smoking before surgery
- You are not concerned with a completely natural-looking or -feeling breast

- You are not concerned about loss of sensation
- You do not want or can't have flap reconstruction
- You are willing to accept that you may need to remove and replace implants in the future

Who Is Not a Good Candidate for Implants?

- You are pregnant and/or plan to breastfeed in the future
- You are a smoker and don't wish to quit
- You want new breasts that look and feel 100 percent natural
- You want to maintain as much sensation as possible
- You prefer the idea of using your own tissue for reconstruction

Pros and Cons of Breast Reconstruction with Implants

Pros

- Implants have been done for a long time, and most plastic surgeons are experienced in using them
- They can look very natural if done correctly
- Implants can improve the look of your natural breasts if they were not proportional to the body, symmetrical, or the lacked volume or tone you like
- Implants done in conjunction with a breast lift can correct large, drooping breasts (called ptosis of the breast)

Cons

- Breast implants may need to be replaced in the future
- Implants may rupture or cause infections and pain that require their removal and replacement
- Done incorrectly, implants may slip out of place or move around
- Scar tissue may form around the implant, hardening or misshaping the breast, which requires surgery to fix
- Rippling may occur if the surgeon uses textured implants

- Occasionally the internal pockets for the implants are placed too close together so breasts look as though they're joined in the middle, creating a so-called "uniboob" look
- Having implants may make mammograms more difficult to read
- In rare cases, the skin on the breast can erode and the implant show through. This is called *extrusion* and requires surgery.

TYPES OF RECONSTRUCTION WITH BREAST IMPLANTS

There are two methods of reconstruction with implants: immediate reconstruction done at the time of mastectomy (also referred to as one-step, direct-to-implant, or single stage), and delayed reconstruction with tissue expanders.

Immediate Reconstruction

Immediate reconstruction is becoming more and more popular. In this procedure, the plastic surgeon places a full-size implant at the time of mastectomy, thereby eliminating the need for a second surgery or expansion with a temporary implant. He or she uses an acellular dermal matrix (ADM) like AlloDerm to provide a framework like an internal bra to support the growth of new blood vessels. This sling smoothes the breast contour and holds the implant in place. Thus, the use AlloDerm in concert with your pectoral muscles eliminates the need to create a pocket using a tissue expander, which can require months of discomfort. Some surgeons feel that AlloDerm also reduces pain and the chance of capsular contracture. In addition to AlloDerm, best-known brands of ADM are Tutoplast, DermaMatrix, and Strattice.

Several months after reconstruction, nipple reconstruction and areola tattooing will be done, if desired.

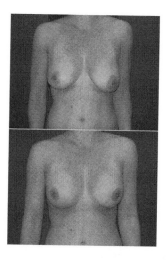

32 year old patient after immediate bilateral breast reconstruction with high profile silicone implant and AlloDerm, by Dr. C. Andrew Salzberg

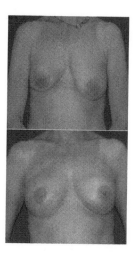

54 year old patient following immediate reconstruction with high profile silicone implant and AlloDerm, by Dr. C. Andrew Salzberg

Who Is a Good Candidate for Immediate Reconstruction?

- You have a tumor that is under 5cm or does not involve the chest wall
- You don't need follow-up chemotherapy or radiation: chemotherapy can affect healing, while radiation can result in unwanted breast changes

- You have not had radiation in the past: irradiated skin is sensitive and less elastic, and may not be able to be stretched adequately to accommodate an implant
- You do not want a second surgery for reconstruction, as in expander reconstruction
- You want to wake up from surgery with a new breast and/or don't want to wait for 6 months to a year for reconstruction to be complete
- You are able to find an experienced, well-regarded surgeon who does one step reconstruction: many surgeons still prefer reconstruction through the expansion process.
- You are willing to have revision surgeries if the first result is not as desired
- You are a C/D cup and want to go a cup smaller and bigger
- You are concerned about the financial aspects of reconstruction. Mastectomy with immediate reconstruction is less expensive than delayed reconstruction; however, this alone should not be a key factor in your decision.
- You want the immediate emotional boost.

Who Is Not a Good Candidate for Immediate Reconstruction?

- You have a large tumor or a tumor that involves the chest wall
- You have already had radiation for breast cancer (with some exceptions)
- You are not sure you want reconstruction at this time
- You cannot find an experienced surgeon in your area trained in one-step reconstruction
- You do not want to have possible revision surgeries in the future
- You have a thin or compromised mastectomy flap

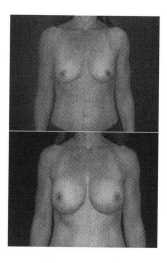

47 year old patient following immediate bilateral breast reconstruction with high profile silicone implant and AlloDerm, by Dr. C. Andrew Salzberg

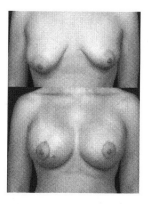

21 year old female following bilateral nipple sparing mastectomy with immediate reconstruction with tissue expander, AlloDerm and injection of Botox into the pectoralis major muscle. Reconstruction completed with subsequent placement of Natrelle Style 45 round silicone implants and bilateral circumareolar mastopexy and fat injection. By Dr. Allen Gabriel.

Pros of Immediate Reconstruction

- Only one surgery needed for mastectomy and breast reconstruction.
- Immediate reconstruction eliminates the need for the tissue expansion process, which can be time-consuming and uncomfortable.

- The breast mound is in place immediately following mastectomy, which may help reduce emotional stress and enhance positive body image.
- Complication rates are lower overall compared with two-stage implant-based reconstruction.

Cons

- There is a higher risk of skin necrosis (cell injury that result in the death of tissue), and implant loss compared with delayed reconstruction.
- It has many of the risks associated implant-based reconstruction, including infection, implant extrusion, implant rupture, implant malposition, capsular contracture, and rippling.
- It requires the surgeon to have specialized training.
- Immediate reconstruction may require more than one step. You may need additional outpatient revision surgeries to correct symmetry as implants settle in.

Delayed Reconstruction (Reconstruction with Tissue Expanders)

With delayed reconstruction, the actual breast reconstruction is completed through a series of four steps that occur over a period of six months or so, and result in permanent breast implants. It is an excellent option if you want to create a placeholder for a future reconstruction or if you want to change or augment the size of your breast. Here is how it works.

1. The first step in many delayed reconstructions is the insertion of a place-holding, temporary implant called a tissue expander on top of your chest muscles during mastectomy to create a pocket for the permanent implant. An expander is like balloon that is filled with saline over several months to help stretch the muscle and create the correct size pocket for the shape and size of your permanent implant, which is inserted later. Please remember: expanders allow you the opportunity to reshape or resize your breasts. Many surgeons assume women

want bigger breasts with implants, but it is your choice! Remember to speak up about what you want and to see before and after photos of both augmented and reduced breasts.

2. To gradually fill the expander, your surgeon will place a magnetic port within the expander (usually at the bottom of the breast) that can be accessed through the skin. The surgeon will inject sterile saline into the expander through this port immediately and then every two or so weeks. Although your new breast may not have a nipple or areola, the expander gives the immediate appearance of a little mound, which may be a psychological boost. In fact, the expander process is quite remarkable! With each fill you'll see significant improvement in the shape and size of your new breasts.

3. During the final one or two fills, your surgeon will overinflate the expander to stretch the skin and make sure there is enough to cover the implant when it is exchanged, as well as achieve aesthetically pleasing results.

4. You will have surgery to replace the temporary expander with a permanent implant of your choice.

5. During the expansion process, you'll wear a surgical bra and later can wear your regular bras once they fit. Be prepared to make some adjustments to your wardrobe during the expansion progress. The Makeup and Style chapter shows you how. In general, if you use the tissue expander method, the entire process from mastectomy to completely reconstructed breast is one year.

Reconstruction Timeline

1. Expanders are inserted during mastectomy surgery.

2. Every few weeks or so over the next six to eight weeks, the surgeon will inject additional fluid into the expander. These fill appointments are quick and usually painless, but sometimes cause aching afterward due to the stretching process. Your surgeon will also work with you to schedule your fills in conjunction with any chemotherapy you may be receiving.

3. When both you and your surgeon are happy with size and volume of the breast, and symmetry is accomplished, the tissue expander will be removed and the surgeon will do "exchange surgery." He or she will remove the expander and insert an implant under the chest muscle, where the expander had been. If you have a unilateral mastectomy, the surgeon will probably do a breast lift, reduction, implant, or other cosmetic procedure to the nonaffected breast to achieve symmetry. Exchange surgery is considered simple, and it is often performed as an outpatient procedure. Be prepared to be sore and swollen for a few weeks while you heal.

4. Nipple reconstruction (if desired) is done usually at least three months after healing; however, it can also be done at any time in the far future. See below.

5. Nipple and areola tattooing (if desired) is done usually at least six months after nipple reconstruction. See below.

Who Is a Good Candidate for Delayed Reconstruction?

- Your skin and chest muscles are tight and flat so that one-step reconstruction is not an option
- You have poor circulation in the chest area or poor wound healing in the past
- You have had previous radiation
- You are OK with waiting six months for your new breasts to be completed
- You are just not sure you want to reconstruct now or you have not decided what type of reconstruction you would like (implant vs. flap).
- You have time in your schedule to go to biweekly fill appointments

Who Is Not a Good Candidate for Delayed Reconstruction?

- You have had radiation in the past: irradiated skin is sensitive and less elastic and may not be able to be stretched adequately to accommodate an implant
- You have a history of poor circulation in the chest area or poor wound healing in the past

Pros

- Expanders allow you time to make decisions about what type of reconstruction you want. An expander can make it possible to have either implants *or* tissue reconstruction.
- You may want to give yourself the time to mourn the loss of your natural breasts. Some women feel that direct-to-implant does not allow time to process what has happened.
- Aesthetic results can be excellent, and the time expanders take allow you to fine-tune the shape and size of your breasts.
- If done correctly, follow-up surgeries to correct asymmetry and other issues may not be necessary.

Cons

- Reconstruction with expanders takes time. If you want to wake up from your mastectomy with whole, new breasts, this method is not for you.
- If you are only reconstructing one breast, be prepared to be lopsided while the expander is inflated.
- You may need to change your style of clothing or wear a prosthesis during the process.
- Skin and muscle stretching between fills can be uncomfortable.

Flap Reconstruction Procedures

The other form of breast reconstruction is called tissue flap. There are many variations, but they all share the same principle: use of your own tissue, including skin, muscle and fat, taken from another part of your body to rebuild the breast. The place where the tissue is taken is called the donor site and is usually the abdomen (exceptions and techniques are discussed below).

After your initial surgery in which the tissue from the donor site is placed in the breast area to create a new breast, a "revision surgery" is often needed after the reconstructed breast settles in. Additional shaping with fat liposuctioned from the donor site (or elsewhere) to achieve symmetry and "lift" is commonplace, as are procedures that minimize existing scars.

Finally, nipple and areola reconstruction and tattooing will be done once any revision surgeries are finished.

All flap procedures require significant surgical skill, and the operation and healing are much longer than with implant reconstruction (six to twelve weeks for initial surgery). In addition to two immediate surgeries and a second scar at the donor site, you may require a later revision to create an aesthetically appealing result.

Who Is a Good Candidate for a Flap Reconstruction?

- You do not want breast implants
- You do not mind having two scars: on on your breast and the second at the donor site
- You would like to have body-contouring surgery as part of the reconstruction process (see below)
- You want to retain as much sensation as possible
- You want your breasts to change naturally as you age or lose/gain weight
- You live in an area with surgeons especially trained in flap reconstruction

Who Is Not a Good Candidate for Flap Reconstruction?

- You do not care if your reconstructed breast is made from your own tissue and want a less complex surgery
- You would like the look and feel of breast implants
- You want to change the size and shape of your breast radically. Implants can offer more choices.
- You do not have the time for the additional pain and healing

Pros of Flap Procedures

- You can rebuild breasts from your own body rather than implants.
- The breast is more natural looking and will act like a natural breast.
- The breast will gain and lose weight with the rest of your body.
- You may regain sensation that you would not with implant reconstruction.

- Reconstructing the breast with your own tissue may be an emotional boost.
- There is no prolonged tissue expansion process.
- Matching the other breast, if desired, is easier.
- The procedure can act as mini-liposuction at the belly, hips, abdomen, back, or love-handles area.
- The procedure can be performed even with tissue compromised by previous radiation.
- The procedure can be used to fix a lumpectomy defect.
- It is permanent and will not require replacement, as implants eventually may.

Cons

- Surgery and healing will be longer (generally six to twelve weeks), particularly if you're having chemotherapy at the same time.
- You will experience pain during healing at donor site and breast area: basically, you are recovering from two operations at the same time.
- There will be possible additional expense: flap procedures are more complicated procedures than implants.
- You may have trouble achieving perfect symmetry if you opt to reconstruct only the affected breast.
- Lumps can form in the reconstructed breast.
- You may have muscle weakness and numbness at the donor site.
- Your normal range of motion may be compromised.
- You will have a second scar at the donor site.
- With the TRAM flap, hernia and bulging may occur.
- You may have fluid collection (seroma).
- You may have necrosis on the reconstructed breast due to insufficient blood supply.
- It may be difficult to find a surgeon in your area: these procedures require additional training and a high level of skill.

Types of Flap Procedures

There are many types of flap procedures. Here are the basic types and how they are performed.

TRAM [transverse rectus abdominis myocutaneous] Flap

The TRAM flap was, until recently, the most common form of tissue reconstruction even though it has largely been replaced by the DIEP flap (see below).

A TRAM flap basically transfers skin, fat, and muscle from the lower abdominal region through a horizontal incision across the hips. The procedure does leave a visible scar, but this can usually be covered by underwear or a bathing suit. The TRAM flap also removes muscle from the abdominal wall and might compromise strength. Nonetheless, it can yield excellent results in the hands of an experienced, as our images show, and can also reduce excess abdominal fat.

There are three types of TRAM flaps: pedicled, free flap and muscle-sparing TRAM.

- In a pedicled TRAM flap, the surgeon rotates the flap of tissue taken from your abdomen and moves it through a tunnel of skin and fat to the chest. The surgeon then shapes it into a breast mound and sutures it into place.
- In the more complex free flap TRAM reconstruction, the skin, fat, and muscle are completely detached and moved to the chest wall. The tissue is then reattached through microsurgery.
- Muscle-sparing TRAM is similar to the free flap TRAM, but leaves more of the abdominal muscles intact.

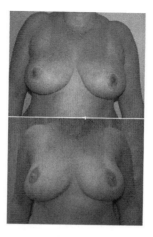

Bilateral breast reconstruction with immediate pedicled
TRAM flaps, by Dr. Danielle DeLuca-Pytell

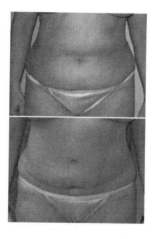

TRAM reconstruction: Abdomen of the same patient after bilateral
pedicled TRAM reconstruction, by Dr. Danielle DeLuca-Pytell

Who Is a Good Candidate for a TRAM Flap?

- You have sufficient abdominal fat to create the breast mound
- You have not had previous abdominal surgery (caesarian section may be an exception)
- You won't mind a horizontal scar and potential altered appearance of your belly button
- Your lifestyle allows you time to heal completely (six to twelve weeks)

- You want to maintain sensation in your reconstructed breast as much as possible
- You would like a tummy tuck as part of the reconstruction process

Who Is Not a Good Candidate for a TRAM flap?

- You are thin and do not have sufficient abdominal fat to build a breast
- You have had previous abdominal surgery (caesarian section may be an exception)
- You do not want a scar or potentially altered belly button
- You do not have time to heal from the process

Pros

- It is a tried-and-true reconstruction technique and may be the only available to you.
- It gives an additional little tummy tuck with your reconstruction.
- Clothing easily hides the scar.
- Results can be very natural.

Cons

- It can weaken abdominal walls, sometimes permanently.
- It will leave a visible horizontal scar.
- It can alter the appearance of your belly button.
- It takes a long time to heal.
- It may produce a hernia.

DIEP (deep inferior epigastric perforator) Flap

The DIEP flap can be thought of the new-and-improved TRAM flap. It is the most sophisticated flap surgery currently performed.

Like a TRAM flap, a DIEP flap uses skin, tissue, an artery, and a vein attached to your tissue flap to supply blood to the flap when it is transplanted to your chest. Unlike a TRAM flap, however, a DIEP flap *does not* remove or transfer the muscle. Instead, it takes the necessary blood vessels from beneath the muscle and reattaches them in the chest. Sensory nerve reconstruction may also be performed at the time. This allows for improved long-term sensation in the reconstructed breast.

Sometimes a patient does not have enough abdominal tissue to do a traditional DIEP flap. In this case, a surgeon may perform a "stacked" DIEP flap. In this variant, two individual flaps of tissue are taken from both sides of the abdomen and stacked on top of each other to create a larger breast.

Because the DIEP flap leaves the abdominal muscles intact, recovery time and pain are lessened. It gives the same aesthetic results as a traditional TRAM.

DIEP flaps are now often preferred over TRAM flaps because they preserve more abdominal strength. They can also be less painful and have a shorter recovery time (two to four weeks instead of the six to twelve weeks with TRAM). However, DIEP flaps are complicated microsurgeries, and finding a surgeon who does them regularly is imperative to achieve good results.

> *DIEP flaps are sometimes referred to as muscle-sparing flaps. Dr. Ariel N. Rad explains: "This is a highly complex microsurgical operation whereby the abdominal skin and fat (not muscle!) is carefully removed and then transferred to the breast where the blood vessels are connected under a microscope with tiny sutures that are thinner than a human hair. Patients also have a tummy tuck in the process, which is a bonus!"*

Who Is a Good Candidate for a DIEP Flap?

- You have not had previous abdominal surgery, including a hysterectomy, tubal ligation, or gallbladder surgery (c-section is sometimes OK)
- You have sufficient abdominal fat
- You are a nonsmoker
- You are age sixty-five or under
- Your lifestyle requires quicker and less painful healing time
- You do not plan to get pregnant
- You would like a tummy tuck as part of reconstruction

Who Is Not a Good Candidate for a DIEP Flap?
- You have had previous abdominal surgery, including a hysterectomy, tubal ligation, or gallbladder surgery (c-section is sometimes OK)
- You plan to get pregnant
- You are thin, do not have adequate abdominal fat or wish to have a tummy tuck
- You are a smoker
- You are sixty-five or older
- You have diabetes or other circulatory disease
- You live in an area where a surgeon trained in DIEP will be difficult to find

Pros
- You will have the same aesthetic results as having a TRAM flap but with less downtime.
- It is possible to enlarge breasts if surgeon performs stacked DIEP.
- The procedure can offer a significant tummy tuck.
- Clothing can easily hide scars.
- You will retain abdominal strength.
- It is less painful than having a TRAM flap.
- There is less risk of a hernia than in having a TRAM flap.

Cons
- The surgery is very complicated, and performing it requires extensive training. You may have a difficult time finding a surgeon in your area.
- It can still weaken abdominal walls.
- It leaves a visible horizontal scar on belly.
- It can alter the appearance of your belly button.
- The tissue flap may die if reconstruction fails. In this case, it will have to be removed.

SIEA (superficial inferior epigastric artery) Flap

A variation of the DIEP flap is the SIEA flap, which uses tissue from the *lower* abdomen to reconstruct the breast. It is different from the DIEP because it does not require taking blood vessels going through or around the abdominal muscles. Rather, the blood vessels are taken from the fatty tissue beneath the skin of the lower belly without moving the muscle. As with a DIEP flap, this leaves the muscle intact, and abdominal strength is preserved. Sensory nerve reconstruction may also be performed. Recovery time is usually four to six weeks.

The SIEA flap is much less frequently performed since the arteries in most patients are generally too small to sustain the flap. Only 15 to 20 percent of patients have the anatomy required to allow this procedure. Unfortunately, it is not possible to determine this before surgery. Also, a SIEA flap usually creates smaller breasts and can have blood-flow problems.

Who Is a Good Candidate for a SIEA Flap?
- See DIEP Flap above

Who Is Not a Good Candidate for a SIEA Flap?
- See DIEP flap above
- Your breasts are large and you want to stay that size

Pros
- See pros DIEP flap above.
- There is little risk of a hernia.
- The procedure has a less than 1 percent failure rate.

Cons
- See cons of DIEP flap.
- It cannot be used to create a large breast.
- There is a higher rate of blood-flow problems, which can produce lumps.
- It may cause a hernia.

LAT (latissimus dorsi) Flap
In a LAT flap, skin and fat are taken from the back muscles (latissimus dorsi) and surrounding fat of the back often referred to as "lats." These are

the largest muscles in your body and allow coverage for large wounds that are sometimes associated with modified or radical mastectomy surgery.

This technique is not commonly performed except in the case of radical mastectomies, on women who are very thin or have had radiation to the abdomen or other donor sites. A LAT flap leaves two significant scars: one on your back and the other on your breast. Your surgeon can preferentially place the back scar so it is hidden by your bra. This procedure may compromise muscle functioning in your back.

A LAT flap is sometimes used in conjunction with an implant to reconstruct the breast. It may offer good results, and recovery may be shorter than with other flap techniques. It can also be used to cover a lumpectomy defect.

A new variant of the LAT flap, the TDAP (thoracodorsal artery perforator) flap, uses tissue harvested from the same region as the LAT flap, but does not sacrifice muscle. It is sometimes used to supplement a LAT or other flap and provide additional volume.

There are downsides to the LAT flap, and not everyone is a good candidate. It can cause asymmetry in the back, a sizable scar, and possible denting where muscle was removed. Additionally, the color and texture of the skin on your back different than your chest skin, so there may be a visible difference.

Who Is a Good Candidate for a LAT Flap?
- You have had previous abdominal surgery or abdominal radiation
- You are nervous and want a procedure with a low rate of complications
- You have excess back fat but little abdominal fat
- You want to cover a lumpectomy defect
- You have had a failed TRAM or DIEP reconstruction or are not a candidate for them
- You plan to become pregnant
- You have had previous radiation
- A breast implant may not be large enough to match the opposite breast
- You don't mind having a back scar

- You have small to medium breasts
- You are not excessively active and would not be affected by the partial loss of an important muscle group
- You live in an area where you can't have a TRAM or DIEP flap

Who Is Not a Good Candidate for a LAT Flap?
- You have had previous chest surgery or abdominal surgery
- You do not want to end up with two scars
- You are very active and the loss of movement and weakness in your back would be a problem
- You have large breasts and do not want implants in addition to tissue transfer
- You are uncomfortable with having your back as a donor site
- You have diabetes or other circulatory disease

Pros
- It is a good option for a thin woman who does not want implant reconstruction.
- It can remove excess back fat.
- It can cover a lumpectomy defect.
- You have large breasts and a breast implant alone may not match the natural breast.
- The complication rate is low.

Cons
- You will have two large, visible scars.
- Back muscles will be compromised or even partially lost, with impaired mobility.
- You may possibly need an implant too.
- Because this is specialized surgery, you may have trouble finding a surgeon.

GAP (gluteal artery perforator) Flaps

A GAP flap uses tissue from your buttocks area to reconstruct the breast. Gluteal tissue has a similar density and feel as natural breasts and can form a very natural but firm breast. Furthermore, you will not lose muscle function.

If you are very slender and therefore not a good candidate for a TRAM or DIEP flap, or previous implants have failed, you may still have enough gluteal tissue for a GAP flap. However, GAP flaps are very complex surgeries, and it may be difficult to find a surgeon in your area. In fact, GAP procedures are infrequently performed due to their complexity and length of time (eight to ten hours). Finally, they are usually not recommended for patients wanting bilateral reconstruction because the risk of complications rises.

There are three variants of the GAP flap.

- The SGAP (superior gluteal artery perforator) uses tissue from the upper love-handles region where hips meets the buttocks to create the flap. This can be a good for women who have an excess of fat there, but may also flatten the buttocks.
- The LSGAP (superior lumbosacral gluteal artery perforator) is a more sophisticated version of the SGAP. It is sometimes referred to as the cushion flap. This technique uses tissue from the waist down and allows a portion of the love-handles region to be used *without* distorting the buttocks. Unlike other GAP flaps, this procedure allows a bilateral reconstruction at the same time, and recovery time is quicker.
- The IGAP (inferior gluteal artery perforator) harvests tissue from the lower buttocks area through an incision made in the crease where the buttocks meets the thigh. It is sometimes called the in-the-crease flap. Although this procedure leaves a minimal, easily hidden scar, it can also result in a flattened bottom with loss of significant volume.

Who Is a Good Candidate for a GAP Flap?
- You do not have adequate abdominal fat for a TRAM or DIEP flap
- You have had previous abdominal surgery

- You are active and are not a good candidate for a LAT flap
- You would like a butt and thigh lift
- You have only one breast to reconstruct
- You would like a scar that is virtually hidden
- You have sagging or ample buttocks
- You would like a firmer, more youthful-looking breast than one from an abdominal flap
- You live in an area with expert surgeons who do this lesser-performed procedure

Who Is Not a Good Candidate for a GAP Flap?

- You have had previous liposuction in the buttocks and thigh area
- You have had previous abdominal or back surgery
- You are very thin and do not have adequate gluteal tissue
- You have diabetes or other circulatory disease
- You would like to have both breasts reconstructed
- An experienced surgeon is not available in your area

Pros

- It can produce firm, very natural-feeling breasts.
- The procedure offers a butt lift and possible significant body recontouring.

Cons

- The surgery is very complex, requiring additional training.
- It may recontour the body in a nonpleasing manner.
- Recovery time is significant.
- It may produce large, visible scar.

TUG (transverse upper gracilis) Flap

A TUG flap uses thigh muscle for reconstruction. It is a relatively new process using skin, fat, and muscle in the gracilis (midthigh), which can give enough tissue for an A/B cup. It is particularly useful if a woman does not have adequate abdominal or buttocks tissue for an abdominal/GAP flap, or has had previous abdominal surgeries. A TUG flap leaves a minimal scar near the groin area and little deformation to the area. Surprisingly, this procedure does not affect the look of the leg or its function, but you may see a 10 to 50 percent reduction in original breast size. Depending on your preferences, this can be a good or bad thing. It also offers an inner-thigh lift and has a low rate of complications.

A TUT (transverse upper-thigh flap) is a variant of GAP, and uses tissue from the upper-thigh region. It best for women with excess thigh tissue. This procedure carries with it the bonus of significant thigh contouring or reduction if liposuction is performed at the same time. Like a TUG flap, it spares muscle.

Who Is a Good Candidate for a TUG/TUT Flap?
- You have adequate fat in your thighs
- You'd like inner-thigh contouring or reduction
- You are not a good candidate for other flap procedures because of diabetes or other circulatory disease
- You have already had a tummy tuck or other abdominal surgery
- You wish to have small to medium breast reconstruction

Who Is Not a Good Candidate for a TUG/TUT flap?
- You are slender and do not have adequate thigh tissue
- You wish to have medium to large breast reconstruction (large B cup size and up)
- You do not wish to have a scar in your groin region

Pros
- It recontours the thigh region.
- It creates a small, firm breast.
- It leaves a very small scar.

Cons
- The surgery is complex.

LAP (lumbar artery perforator) Flap

The LAP flap uses soft tissue from the region just above the buttocks (love handles) to reconstruct the breast. It also allows a larger breast to be reconstructed.

This procedure spares muscle and can significantly recontour the hip and buttocks area. It leaves a scar at waist level that clothing can hide. It may be a good choice if DIEP and LAT flaps are not an option.

Who Is a Good Candidate for a LAP Flap?

- You are not able to have an abdominal flap
- You have excess fat in the upper buttocks region and would like to recontour
- You want to have larger breasts than you can with a DIEP or GAP flap
- You will not mind a large horizontal scar

Who Is Not a Good Candidate for a LAP Flap?

- You are very slender and do not have adequate tissue in the region
- You do not wish to have a large scar

Pros

- Harvesting the tissue is easy and does not interfere with muscle.
- It can offer a significant butt lift and love handles contouring.
- It can give more volume than a TUG/TUT flap.

Cons

- It will leave a large horizontal scar.

Body Lift Flap

The Body Lift flap is a very new procedure that harvests tissue from both the buttocks area and waistline, allowing breasts to have maximum volume at the same time as significantly recontouring the waist and buttocks area. It essentially does breast reconstruction, a tummy tuck, *and* butt lift at the same time. At the time of publication, Body Lift reconstruction is performed at only one or two facilities.

NIPPLE RECONSTRUCTION

Modern reconstruction procedures can produce beautiful, natural breasts. However, unless you have had nipple-sparing surgery, most procedures remove the nipple and areola in the process. It is your choice to decide if you'd like to have new ones created. Some women are perfectly satisfied to have breast mounds that look natural in clothing and just have new nipples tattooed. Others wish to have the most natural look with tangible nipples. The choice is entirely personal.

Nipple reconstruction is usually scheduled three months after reconstructive surgery and is sometimes done during any revision reconstruction surgery after the initial healing. Waiting until this date allows the breast time to heal and settle into place so the nipple can be placed in an aesthetically pleasing manner, and you can always wait to have nipples reconstructed at a later date. Insurance should cover the procedure as part of the reconstruction process.

Reconstructed nipples will not have the sensation or movement of natural nipples. However, beautiful results are totally possible and may outweigh the loss of natural nipples you may feel. As with any reconstructive process, you can decide how big you would like your new nipples to be, how much projection they will have, and, if you are having a nipple tattoo, how dark or light it will be.

Two kinds of nipple reconstruction techniques are commonly used. The first is nipple reconstruction from a flap of breast skin. The second method uses skin grafts from the inner thigh (or sometimes ear, groin, or buttocks) to build a new nipple. Areola reconstruction is usually done with a skin graft from the abdomen.

Building a Nipple from a Flap of Skin

In this procedure, small pieces of skin from the reconstructed breast are used to build a nipple. Your surgeon will create a flap by cutting and lifting skin from the reconstructed breast and twist or fold it into cone shape. This creates a little bump, which is then sutured to create a nipple mound with volume and projection like a natural nipple.

Nipple flaps can produce good volume, but are sometimes augmented with skin substitutes like AlloDerm or natural cartilage to give them a firmer core. This procedure allows for more projection, especially with patients who have undergone tissue expansion that has thinned the skin.

Most flap nipple reconstruction are done in the same way, but differ in the shape of the incision used to lift the skin and recreate the nipple. Usually these are the skate flap (most widely used), star flap, CV flap, arrow flap, bell flap, etc. The skate flap seems to cause the least alteration of the shape of the breast contour.

Nipples created from flap techniques will shrink during the first year and deflate, so don't be alarmed when your surgeon creates a nipple that is larger and "pointier" than you expected. Sometimes your surgeon will use fat grafts or fillers such as Juvederm or Restylane to increase nipple projection if the nipple does deflate too much. This can also be done at a later date when nipples have a chance to naturally flatten and conform to the breast.

Areola reconstruction is usually performed a few months after nipple reconstruction.

Nipples built with flap reconstruction will not have any pigment (color) except for whatever scarring there may be. Most women opt for nipple tattooing to create the color and details of a natural nipple (see below).

Pros

- Nipple flap reconstruction uses only one incision and therefore produces one scar, which can be camouflaged by subsequent tattooing.
- Nipple will have natural movement.
- Nipple should have good volume and projection.

Cons

- Nipple may deflate more than desired.
- It leaves a scar that may or may not be camouflaged by tattooing.
- May require a fat graft or filler to enhance projection.
- Additional tattooing may be needed to achieve a natural appearance.

Building a Nipple from a Skin Graft

In this procedure, the surgeon removes a piece of skin from the inner thigh or groin region to create the nipple mound. Hair follicles will be removed, and the surgeon will then remove the top layer of skin from the nipple area of the reconstructed breast and attach the graft in its place. Sometimes skin to be grafted is taken from the ear, eyelid, or buttocks, but inner thigh or groin tissue is most often used because of its similarity in color and texture to natural nipples.

Nipple grafts can offer excellent projection and, if they are made from groin skin, a natural look. Some women worry about whether using skin from this area will leave them with hairy nipples. This is not the case: hair follicles have been removed prior to surgery, and if it does indeed happen, most of the time just a single hair or two will crop up.

It must be noted that the incision from the donor site of the graft reconstruction can be painful, especially if it is in the groin region.

Pros

- Nipple will have better volume and projection than in flap nipple reconstruction.
- The chance of deflation is much less.
- Nipple may have a natural look without needing additional tattooing.

Cons

- There is a secondary surgical site and therefore a second scar.
- Graft failure, in which skin is not grafted to the nipple area with an adequate blood supply and therefore fails, is possible.
- A hair or two may grow on nipples if not all follicles are removed. Electrolysis can help.

NIPPLE AND AREOLA TATTOOING

In about eight to twelve weeks, or after your nipple has healed, you are ready for nipple tattooing if you desire. Note that nipple-areola complex tattooing goes by a number of names: repigmentation, NAC tattooing, micropigmentation, etc. We use the term *nipple tattooing* to keep it simple.

Not everyone wants to go through one more procedure at this point, but for many women nipple tattooing is the proverbial icing on the cake. It marks the end of the reconstruction journey and adds the final realistic touch. For many women, this simple procedure helps them reclaim their femininity... and life.

Your plastic surgeon may offer to tattoo your nipples for you. We generally do not recommend this! It is very important to have your nipple tattoo done by a professional tattoo artist experienced in 3-D tattooing. Plastic surgeons are experts at the operating table, and while some are very good at creating realistic nipples, others are not. If you are thinking of having your surgeon do your nipple tattoos, *you must ask for before and after photos.*

On the other hand, a tattoo artist experienced in nipple and areola tattooing can mimic the projection, shape of the areola, and natural texture of the nipple. Professional tattoo artists can recreate the most natural, 3-D-looking nipple—right down to the Montgomery glands surrounding the areola. Artists will use "painterly" techniques to achieve naturalistic highlighting and color variation. They can make the nipple look like it's protruding a bit and hide any scarring you may have.

Nipple tattooing is not a one-step process in most cases. Expect to have at least two to three visits, spread out over time, to achieve the color and look you want. The second visit is usually about four weeks after the first. And you will need color touch-ups any time from one to five years after.

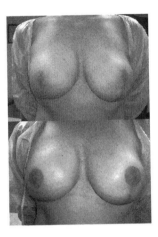

Bilateral nipple tattoo, by Dr. Laura Reed

Safety

Because tattooing is a technique that breaks the surface of the skin with a needle and introduces colored ink, infection and other problems are always a possibility. Most tattoo artists use sterilized needles; however, this alone will not prevent cross-contamination from the tattoo artist's hand (which should be gloved) to other surfaces. Proper disinfection and sterilization needs to be done to prevent the spread of pathogens and bacteria.

Paramedical tattoo artist Dr. Laura Reed explains: Artists can use different types of equipment including digital computerized machines, rotary analog machines, manual devices (for the hand-tapping method), or traditional coil machines (used for conventional body art). Regardless of the type of equipment used, all artists utilize various tattoo needles to implant the pigment(s) into the middle layer of the patient's skin called the dermis. The upper layer of skin (epidermis) will be 'broken' and opened to the extent that body fluids (blood and/or lymph) will travel to the surface. Therefore, while the artist is working, her/his gloved hands, the needle and machine hand piece, pigment cups, etc. will be touching that patient's skin and body fluids. Those body fluids might contain microorganisms called blood-borne pathogens, and that is where the risk for cross contamination exists. It is imperative that *all* tattoo artists fully know and understand exactly what to do—and what not to do—to prevent or minimize body fluids from touching and contaminating surfaces. They must also know how to properly protect and disinfect surfaces that cannot be sterilized. They must know how to correctly sterilize any non-disposable items that may be used and also know how to properly maintain their sterilization devices such as an autoclave. Autoclaves must be periodically tested using an outside lab to ensure that the correct temperatures are reached for an adequate period of time to completely eradicate all microorganisms and their spores.

"Nationally certified permanent cosmetic professionals and licensed tattoo artists follow strict guidelines established by the Centers for Disease Control (CDC) and Occupational Health and Safety Administration (OSHA). The CDC rules for preventing cross-contamination are extensive. They require thorough education and training to learn all of the detailed steps. The tattooist must then have enough practice in order to prevent mistakes, especially if she/he does not have any medical background." Ask your artist about his or her qualifications.

Choosing your Artist and Facility

Getting a nipple tattoo is quite different than ordinary artistic tattooing and requires more skill. Although it may be tempting to go to a tattoo artist who does beautiful artistic work, it is unlikely that the artist has enough experience in nipple tattooing to give you the best result. Furthermore, a tattoo shop is not the safest or most comfortable site for a tattoo of this sensitive nature.

The most important thing you should do is evaluate the artist's skill and experience in nipple – not just regular – tattooing. Ask about the following issues:

- The facility's Health Department permit should be current, therefore indicating that the equipment and practices meet current standards and have passed inspection.
- Look at before and after photos of the artist's work: before the tattoo, immediately after the tattoo, and once it has healed. It is also helpful to see tattoos that are older to see how they have aged.
- Ask about the artist's training in nipple tattooing.

- Inquire about the frequency of nipple tattooing. An artist may have been doing nipple tattoos for twenty years but may do only one a year!
- Find out how the artist handles pain management, particularly if you want him or her to tattoo both the reconstructed *and* unaffected nipple. While the reconstructed nipple may be numb, the unaffected nipple has full sensation and if can be painful.
- Ask him or her to explain disinfection and sterilization process of any items they use, including autoclaves.
- Get a complete and thorough explanation of the process from start to finish.
- Examine where the tattooing will take place. Ideally it should be in a private, safe, sterile environment used only for medical tattooing. No loud music, distractions, odors, etc.
- Make sure the artist offers a thorough aftercare sheet and instructions.
- Find out when the artist usually does touch-up tattooing.

Pain Management

For some women, the fear of the pain of tattooing alone is enough not to go through with it. Although some artists may brush off the need for pain management or insist it interferes with the ink transfer, an experienced nipple tattoo artist will work with you to make the experience comfortable. Try to remember:

- Your reconstructed nipple is likely to be almost entirely numb!
- Tattoos hurt more on bony parts of the body, like ankles or ribs. A nipple tattoo is done on a fleshy mound, which is naturally less sensitive.
- Your artist can apply a topical numbing agent such as lidocaine to either or both nipples both before *and* during the process. An artist who is a medical professional will even be able to use a prescription-strength product.

Getting the Best Result

The look of your tattoo can be affected by the state of your health in addition to the skill of your artist. Here are some considerations.

Prepare your Skin

Dr. Laura Reed suggests the following to make sure your skin is in the best condition to accept the tattoo:

- If the skin on your reconstructed breast is dry or flaky, a day or two before your appointment, gently apply a facial scrub, rinse, and finish with a good moisturizer.
- If you have elevated scars from reconstructive surgery, consider preliminary microneedling treatments to flatten the scars prior to tattooing.
- Drink extra water: when a woman is well-hydrated, she will not retain water, and swelling during the tattooing process will be less. Cut down on caffeine and avoid alcohol for three to five days before tattooing.
- Reduce the chance of excess bleeding: avoid any blood-thinning medications or supplements (anticoagulants) at least three to five days prior to the tattooing procedure. This includes aspirin (or aspirin-containing products like Alka-Seltzer), NSAIDs (nonsteroidal anti-inflammatories) such as ibuprofen, ginkgo biloba, fish oils, and alcohol.

Consider Bilateral Tattooing

If you have a unilateral reconstruction, you may want to mimic your existing nipple as much as possible. But some tattoo artists work on both nipples to achieve the most realistic result and in doing so enhance the look of the unaffected nipple as well. Nipples can expand, shrink, sag, or change color with age in a way that is unpleasing to you. As with reconstruction, you can now choose the size, shape, color of *both* nipples and areolas with a new tattoo. This is a wonderful opportunity to correct any issues you have with your natural nipple while you create a new one.

If you do want to achieve a perfect balance but don't want to tattoo your unaffected nipple, bring a good photograph of your nipple before surgery.

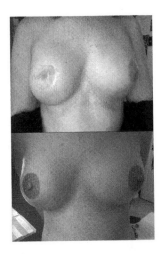

Bilateral nipple tattoo, by Cathi Locati

> "The left areola is often a bit larger than the right one because the breast over the heart is often a bit larger. No two areolas are ever identical."
> —Julie Michaud, micropigmentation expert

Nipple Placement, Size, and Color

Nipple placement is a very important part of achieving a natural result. It may be tempting just to have your artist place them in the center of your breast mounds, but this method can produce tattoos that look fake. Here are a few things to think about and ask your artist about:

- Center the nipple within the *areola* rather than center the areola on the breast mound. No woman's areolas are horizontally straight.
- Talk about whether you want perfectly even or slightly uneven areolas.
- If you were previously unhappy with where your nipple were, "play" with placement to achieve a higher, lower, wider, or narrower look.
- Discuss the size of the areola: you may want to go bigger or smaller than your natural areolas.
- It is easy to make a tattoo larger, but it is difficult to make one smaller. This requires laser or salt removal of part of the tattoo, which can be costly and may not be covered by insurance. Ask your tattoo artist to start with a small sketch and work larger.

- Discuss the colors of the nipple and areola: you may wish to go darker or lighter. The most natural effect will come from a custom blend of colors and the use of much shading. You may be surprised at what colors the artist brings out!

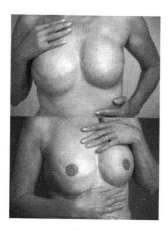

Bilateral nipple tattoo, by Julie Michaud

How It Is Done: Nipple Tattooing Step by Step

Easing the anxiety about a tattoo can be as simple as understanding the process from start to finish. Dr. Laura Reed explains:

"After the areola(s) size, shape, color, and placement have been determined, a topical anesthetic cream or ointment is applied to the breast mound for approximately thirty minutes. I usually mix and prepare the pigments while my patient is numbing, and I also have her read aftercare instructions in case she has any unanswered questions.

"When it is time, the topical anesthetic is wiped off and the templates for the new areolas are drawn. Care is taken to measure correctly for the size we determined beforehand and the placement. Then my patient and I make a visual assessment one last time and make any minor adjustments before the tattooing begins.

"My preference is to have my patients lie down for their procedures. Some artists prefer to have their patients/clients sitting upright or semi-upright (slightly inclined) and believe that is the "right" way. But I believe it is a personal preference. I will follow a template that was drawn with the woman upright, and my patients are satisfied with their results.

"I begin the tattooing process on one breast until it is finished, and then I switch sides. An entire 3-dimensional nipple-areola complex tattoo takes approximately one hour per breast. When completely finished, I immediately take photographs with my patient sitting up or standing. Then I apply antibiotic ointment and a nonstick/nonlatex pad (for example, Telfa) held in place by tape that is suitable for sensitive skin. (Note: Prior to tattooing, "before" photographs are taken, either at the consultation or at some practical point before the final template is drawn.)

"The patient returns for a follow-up procedure (called a touch-up) in approximately six weeks."

What to Expect during Healing

Your tattoo will be sore for the first few days—after all, it is a wound. Here are some other things that may happen during the healing process:

> "In addition to size and color, the woman can decide if she wants perfectly round or slightly uneven areolas. It is not uncommon for women to have egg-shaped areolas. And when they do, they usually 'tilt' inward toward the center of the chest. The woman can also decide if she wants her areolas to have 'defined borders' or a gradient/blurred effect. From a beauty standpoint, it is important for women to know that there is not one 'standard' or 'average' areola in terms of shape, size, or color. They vary as greatly as women's hair color, eye color, and skin tone. To illustrate the vast differences among human female areolas, I show patients several pages from various men's magazines like Playboy and Biker Week that appear to be natural (not airbrushed or altered). That typically elicits a few giggles but proves a valid point."
> —Dr. Laura Reed

- Your tattoo might be darker red, sensitive, and oozy. It is normal to see some of the color wipe off with the oozing.
- As it heals, the surface of the skin may harden. Then it will peel off like a scab or sunburn in about three days, revealing the underlayer. It might itch, but do not pick at it, as this can cause uneven color!

- Your nipple/areola will be darker at first. Don't worry. This will tone down over the next few months to the shade you and your artist chose.

Things to Look Out For

- If your tattoo is very swollen, blistering, giving off pus, or very painful, this might be a sign of infection. Stop using any topical ointments and see your doctor immediately.
- If your tattoo scabs or is healing unevenly, you may lose color in those areas. Call your tattoo artist if excessive scabbing occurs.

Basic Aftercare

A tattoo artist should send you home with a detailed aftercare sheet. Aftercare is important to the success of your tattoo, as improper healing with affect the color and appearance. Follow his or her instructions carefully. Here are some basics from Dr. Laura Reed.

Week One

- Don't touch, cleanse, rub, or otherwise handle your tattoo for at least six hours after it is finished.
- During the first week, you can use cold packs five minutes per hour to bring down any swelling and ease pain.
- If your doctor permits, you might try an antihistamine to bring down redness and tenderness.
- If your doctor permits, you might try Motrin to ease the pain.
- When you do cleanse your tattoo, use a cotton swab with *cool water only*. Avoid hot water and baths.
- Your artist will probably recommend you start using an antibiotic ointment for the first three days. After this, the artist will probably have you switch to another ointment. Please use only what they recommend!
- Use a clean, nonstick pad when you put on a bra or shirt, and. if possible, go braless as much as you can.

Week Two and Beyond
- You can now begin using a gentle cleanser. Your artist will give recommendations.
- Avoid long baths and very hot showers during the second week.
- Avoid sun and tanning. This goes without saying!
- Long periods of time in water are not recommended. This includes pools, lakes, the ocean, etc.
- Use only those skin treatments recommended by your artist.
- For a more detailed aftercare regimen, see FAQ below.

SUN AND TATTOOS. *Sunlight is damaging to tattoos and can result in excessive fading and blurring, as well as increased risk of another cancer. Do not expose your newly tattooed nipple to the sun. Always protect your healed nipples by using sun block on them (along with the rest of your skin.)*

Touch-Ups

All tattoos fade over time, so you will periodically have to have your tattoos touched up to correct color and any blurring that may also occur. Likewise, not all tattoos heal evenly, and you may need color correction a few months down the road. Ask your tattoo artist to write down the formula of your colors so the color can remain consistent.

Scar Camouflage

The common misconception about tattooing to reduce the look of scars is that it does not work. However, depending on the placement, type of skin, and type of scar, it is very possible to mask the scar beautifully. Please refer to the "Scar Treatment" chapter.

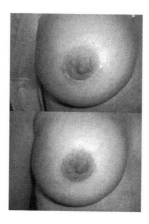

Tattoo camouflage of areola scar, by Dr. Laura Reed

FREQUENTLY ASKED QUESTIONS ABOUT BREAST RECONSTRUCTION

Does getting flap breast reconstruction increase my risk for reoccurring cancer?
Dr. Ariel N. Rad: "The answer is emphatically no! In a meta-analysis study of 1,444 mastectomies, no relationship was found between local recurrence of breast cancer after mastectomy and reconstruction. In other words, having reconstruction does not increase a woman's risk of developing a recurrence of cancer.

"Furthermore, using your own tissue for breast reconstruction does not affect the detection and treatment of local recurrence of breast cancer. The transplanted tissue (whether from the abdomen or back) does not turn into breast tissue; it stays as the same tissue and thus has zero risk of developing breast cancer. If a recurrence of breast cancer happens, it's due to cancer cells being left behind after the mastectomy or the fact that the cancer has already spread to the lymph nodes. However, this is quite rare."

I'm concerned that breast reconstruction may not be safe.

Dr. Ariel N. Rad: "Breast reconstruction is generally safe. As with any surgery, there are risks associated with the operation and with anesthesia, and these relate to how many medical illnesses a patient has.

"Heart disease, lung, kidney, or arterial disease, tendency for developing blood clots ('deep venous thrombosis,' or DVT), etc. are all major risk factors for significant complications during anesthesia. Risk factors for plastic surgery relate to a patient's ability to heal wounds. Aside from this, other risks of breast surgery include asymmetry and scars—while it is the plastic surgeon's goal to create perfect symmetry and minimize scars, everyone heals differently, so it's hard to predict."

How have lumpectomy surgeries changed since the potentially disfiguring ones of the past?

Dr. John P. Rimmer: "The old style of lumpectomy incision was to go through fatty tissue, cut out a lump of tissue, and then close the skin, as in a biopsy. This leaves a space that fills with fluid as it heals. The area can collapse and fill with scar tissue, therefore getting distorted. Now we try to close with tissue moved from another part of breast, as in used in mammoplasty.

"We can now remove about 20 percent breast volume with a reasonable cosmetic result. Lumpectomy should be done when the surgeon can get the cancer out, achieve a good aesthetic outcome, and retain a good-looking breast.

"If you're doing a lumpectomy, there should be no consideration of plastic surgery because of the new concept of oncoplastic surgery: a whole catalog of new surgical techniques used to rebuild the breast by a oncoplastic breast surgeon.

"Different women will accept different things in terms of shape of breast. The most important thing is to counsel the patient correctly."

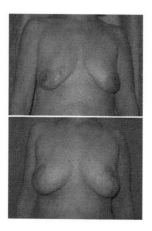

Lumpectomy reconstruction: Immediate left breast reconstruction after lumpectomy with breast reduction pattern, right breast reduction for symmetry, one year following completion of radiation therapy, by Dr. Danielle DeLuca-Pytell

I had a lumpectomy and now have a big dent! What can I do?

Dr. Ariel N. Rad: "A noticeable indentation in the breast as a result of a lumpectomy is challenging to correct, especially after radiation therapy. You may have heard about injection of fat (called fat grafting) into breast tissue to fill in the dent, but this does not work well, particularly if there is radiation damage to the tissues. Transferring healthy tissue with good blood flow to the area is the best way to correct the problem. I would recommend borrowing tissue from the upper back region using a technique called the TDAP flap. The TDAP flap spares the muscle and borrows only the skin and fat."

I have a minor dent from my lumpectomy. I really do not want another surgery! What do you suggest?

Dr. Ariel N. Rad: "If the dent is small, the tissues of your breast are still soft and supple, and there's still good blood flow to the remaining breast tissue, then fat grafting (injection) to the area may improve the indentation without needing a flap operation. This is advantageous, as recovery time is less, additional scars are largely unnecessary, and it's an outpatient operation.

"The limitations of the technique are that only small indentations can be adequately addressed, you may need additional fat grafting procedures to get the final result, and success depends heavily on how healthy the tissues are after radiation."

I have a small lumpectomy defect and would like to reconstruct. Can I achieve symmetry?

The short answer is yes, with implants. See images below and speak with your plastic surgeon.

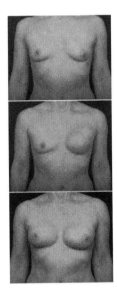

52 year old female presented following left lumpectomy (top pic). She underwent completion of left mastectomy with immediate reconstruction with tissue expander, AlloDerm and injection of Botox into the pectoralis major muscle. (middle pic). She was fully expanded and completed her reconstruction with Natrelle Style 20 round silicone implant on the left and right breast augmentation for matching with Natrelle Style 15. By Dr. Allen Gabriel.

Is immediate reconstruction the wave of the future?

Dr. John P. Rimmer: "I am doing more nipple-sparing mastectomies with immediate reconstruction than before. Although you may need revision surgery down the road or may have a small correction, it has a big psychological benefit to wake up from surgery with a new breast."

I really want immediate reconstruction. But is it right for me?
Dr. C. Andrew Salzberg: "Patients who have already had radiation treatment for breast cancer are not likely candidates for the direct-to-implant procedure. Radiated skin has been compromised, meaning that the blood supply to the breast skin is not as healthy as it was before radiation. A radiated breast can have more trouble healing and is at increased risk for infection if an implant is placed immediately after mastectomy.

"Other patients who may not be good candidates for the direct-to-implant procedure are patients who have very large, pendulous breasts. With this being said, don't worry just yet! We encourage all patients to come in and have a formal consultation where we perform a physical examination as well as review your medical history in detail. We will then be able to determine personalized breast reconstruction options for you."

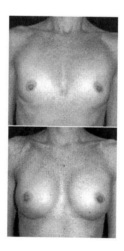

44 year old patient following with bilateral breast reconstruction with shaped implants and AlloDerm, by Dr. C. Andrew Salzberg

Doesn't immediate reconstruction with implants stretch your skin a lot?
Dr. C. Andrew Salzberg, pioneer of the technique, reassures: "Contrary to popular belief, there is no additional expansion or stretching of the skin when placing an implant versus a tissue expander. In order to prove this, we use an advanced imaging technique called the SPY machine while in the operating room. The SPY Elite allows the surgeon to evaluate the perfusion to the skin by using the fluorescent properties of indocyanine green dye (ICG), which is injected intravenously. Video images of blood flow are taken in the operating room, which the surgeon is able to see in real time."

I have a raised, red scar from my mastectomy and plan to get reconstruction. What can I do to help flatten and minimize it?
Before doing anything, see your doctor. Sometimes laser treatments can help. At home you can encourage scar fading by trying cross-fiber or trans-friction massage. Use one or two fingers to gently press and massage your scar perpendicular to the line of the scar. This helps remodel the scar and ensures that the collagen fibers of the scar are aligned properly. At first your scar may appear redder, but as time goes on it will fade noticeably. You can follow the massage with vitamin E oil. Please refer to our Scar Chapter.

I had a unilateral radical mastectomy a long time ago, and am tired of feeling less than whole. Can I still have reconstruction? How might it look?
The short answer is yes. In our photograph below, the patient had implants placed in both breasts along with nipple reconstruction in the affected breast. The results are amazing!

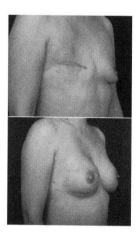

42 year old female following right mastectomy and right breast reconstruction with tissue expander, AlloDerm and injection of Botox into the pectoralis major muscle. She then underwent placement of Natrelle Style 20 round silicone implant on the right and left breast augmentation for matching with Natrelle Style 15 and right nipple areolar reconstruction. By Dr. Allen Gabriel

I'm a smoker. How might this affect my reconstruction?

Dr. Ariel N. Rad: "The most important risk factor [in surgery] is smoking. Nicotine decreases blood flow through the capillaries, the tiny blood vessels that wounds depend on for optimal healing. A review study published this year in the *American Journal of Medicine* showed that nonsmokers had a 41 percent reduction of complications compared with active smokers. For every week of abstinence from smoking, there was a 19 percent reduction of risk, and stopping smoking at least four weeks before surgery was recommended to minimize this risk. I usually advise my patients to stop smoking eight weeks in advance, particularly with larger wounds under tension."

I have had previous radiation and am confused about what reconstructive techniques are OK for me.

Dr. Ariel N. Rad: "Technically, you can have implants after radiation. However, the risk of having problems such as capsular contracture (when the wall of scar around the implant constricts and squeezes the implant, giving the breast a bizarre shape and firm feel) increases significantly after radiation—it happens about 50 to 60 percent of the time. If it develops, capsular contracture may require surgical release of the scar tissue. While this may correct the problem in the short term, the chance of developing capsular contracture again in the future is even higher.

"Other problems associated with radiation and implants include thinning of the breast skin, making an implant more visible or palpable, and having a breast that is 'frozen in time.' This means that that radiated breast doesn't age like the normal unradiated breast, and so over time the breasts would look different. *The definitive solution* for such a problem would be using your own tissue for reconstruction (such as a DIEP flap) and avoiding the use of implants altogether."

I am having a LAT flap, but have heard it can cause a pinched feeling in my armpit and reconstructed breast.
Dr. Ariel N. Rad: "The LAT is a common tissue transfer operation in breast reconstruction. The technique borrows the broad, flat muscle of the upper and middle back (the muscle that gives body builders 'wings') and tunnels it underneath the skin of the armpit to reach the breast.

"Because of this tunneling, it is not uncommon to feel fullness in the armpit—this is the muscle flap passing through the armpit area as it goes to the breast. The sensations usually improve with time as the muscle atrophies, but it may also persist. While somewhat of a nuisance, the important thing is that it's not dangerous to your health.

"Also, it is not unusual to feel contracting sensations in your reconstructed breast after a latissimus dorsi muscle flap. The latissimus muscle is our 'chin-up' muscle. In its native state, it spans the back and attaches to the upper arm bone (the humerus). Unless you're a rock climber, it's rare to do chin-up activities, but certain arm movements may give you the sensation of movement in your breasts. The bottom line is that it won't hurt you."

My implants caused ripples. I am willing to have another surgery, but which one?
Dr. Ariel N. Rad: "Ripples are a difficult problem to correct because there is a very thin layer of tissue (basically just skin) covering the implant. Imagine

a plastic bag half-filled with water; you can see in your mind's eye the wrinkles, ripples, and folds in the bag as the water moves around. Now wrap a wet paper towel around the bag—you can still see the ripples. Now, wrap a thick towel around the bag—the ripples are much less visible because there's more of a layer to hide the wrinkling. The skin layer is like the wet paper towel—it adheres to the implant, and ripples show through. What you really need is an extra thick layer of tissue to hide the ripples, similar to the towel around the bag of water.

"I recommend a tissue transfer operation such as a TDAP or LAT flap. Alternatively, if you have extra fatty tissue in the abdominal or buttock area, removing the implants altogether and performing a DIEP or SGAP flap is a definitive way to get rid of the wrinkles (and the implant altogether) and give the most lasting, natural result."

What are the pros and cons of immediate reconstruction, from a plastic surgeon's standpoint?
Dr. Larry Fan: "Immediate breast reconstruction direct to implant is a newer technique that is growing in popularity. The main advantages of direct to implant reconstruction over a two stage tissue expander reconstruction include:

- Simpler reconstruction with only one surgery needed for mastectomy and breast reconstruction to be performed versus two
- Eliminates the need for the tissue expansion process, which can be time-consuming and uncomfortable
- The breast mound is in place immediately following mastectomy, which may help reduce emotional stress and enhance positive body image
- Probable lower overall complication rates compared to two stage implant based reconstruction
- The main disadvantages of direct to implant reconstruction include:
- Higher risk of skin necrosis and implant loss compared to two stage implant reconstruction

- Not well suited for patients with thin or compromised mastectomy flaps, which usually cannot be determined until in the operating room after the mastectomy is performed
- May have a higher likelihood of requiring an additional revision procedure to optimize breast size and shape
- Still has many of the risks associated implant based reconstruction, including infection, implant extrusion, implant rupture, implant malposition, capsular contracture, and rippling."

I had a lumpectomy a long time ago, and it deformed my breast. Can I still do reconstruction after all this time? And will my insurance cover it?

Dr. Ariel N. Rad: "Yes to both questions. Every woman who undergoes surgery for breast cancer has access to reconstruction—the 1998 Federal Breast Reconstruction Law guarantees this. It also makes provisions for surgical symmetry procedures on the unaffected breast.

"The exact technique…would depend on what your breasts look like, where volume is needed, and how much of a lift or reshaping your breasts require. There are many techniques in a plastic surgeon's armamentarium, so my advice is to be assessed by a board-certified plastic surgeon who routinely performs breast reconstruction."

I want nipple reconstruction but so many women I've spoken to say they really flatten. Any tips on how to minimize this?

Dr. Ariel N. Rad: "The flattening of a reconstructed nipple is one of the frustrating aspects of the technique. A real nipple has a support structure including tiny muscles that allow the nipple to change shape, have projection, and contract. We can only approximate the size and shape of a real nipple, but since non-nipple skin doesn't have the same support structure, it won't last.

"Radiation only makes the situation worse, as the blood flow through the skin has been markedly reduced, and blood flow is key for these operations to succeed. While attempting another nipple reconstruction may be feasible, there is a 100 percent chance that the reconstructed nipple will flatten over time.

"A few techniques can help maintain nipple projection, such as using an injectable dermal filler (like Juvederm or Radiesse); however, these are temporary and will dissolve over six to twelve months."

I am advised to have surgery at a teaching hospital. I'm worried I will not have a choice about my surgeon or if I will be operated on by a doctor in training.
Dr. Ariel N. Rad: "The situation must be assessed individually. At Johns Hopkins [where I practice], we have surgical trainees who are there to assist in surgery and to learn. Their participation is important, as surgeons need assistants to help. [But] rarely do surgeons assign their cases to trainee surgeons. In fact, the attending surgeon is *required* to perform a 'time-out' before the surgery actually begins to ensure that the plan is clear and the operation can commence.

"For peace of mind, you should ask your surgeon directly. When patients ask me, I frankly respond that I am the one performing the surgery with assistants present."

I am choosing implant reconstruction. Will sexual activity and pressure on my breasts cause them to move or burst?
Dr. Ariel N. Rad: "In the first two months after surgery, I generally advise against any direct pressure on breast implants. Beyond two months I feel that infrequent pressure as you describe has no long-term negative impact."

My surgeon wants to use AlloDerm as part of my implant reconstruction. Is this safe?
Dr. C. Andrew Salzberg: "AlloDerm, derived from donated human tissue, is the most studied and widely used acellular dermal matrix. AlloDerm acts as an internal sling/bra to keep the implant in a desirable position as well as protects the delicate skin flap from the silicone implant. It undergoes extensive testing and processing to ensure it is completely stripped of any cellular material."

Is "one step" reconstruction really one step?

Dr. C. Andrew Salzberg: "Although we have nicknamed it the 'one step,' revisions are often needed. As the implants settle and the surrounding breast skin flap heals into place, there are often some minor contour and symmetry irregularities that can be seen. However, these irregularities are easily correctable through an outpatient surgical procedure.

"Patients who are choosing direct to implant to avoid having two separate surgical procedures as with the tissue expander reconstruction should keep in mind that the revision surgery is completely optional and not required. Revision surgeries are done in the ambulatory setting, meaning that the patient can go home the same day and downtime is often minimal."

Health insurance is so confusing these days. How can I be sure I am getting everything I am entitled to?

Kristy Fishman, independent insurance agent and breast cancer survivor: "There are some major medical and surgical benefits that are mandated by federal law. The 1998 Federal Breast Reconstruction Law (also Women's Health and Cancer Rights Act of 1998, or WHRCA) provides the following services, which are covered by health insurance: reconstruction of the breast where the mastectomy was performed; surgery and reconstruction on the other breast to make both breasts symmetrical; and protheses/physical complication (lymphedema) coverage post surgeries. Many resources are available that provide information about your rights and coverage available to you.

"Here are a few informative websites: www.cancer.org, www.cdc.gov, and www.healthcare.gov. Talk to your medical professionals, health insurance broker, insurance plan administrator, and/or your insurance company. Review your policy and understand your benefits that your insurance plan offers."

Can I submit receipts to my insurance company if they are pertinent to my treatment but not automatically covered?

Kristy Fishman: "Keep all receipts and paperwork. Review your plan benefits, summary plan documents (SPD), and/or evidence of coverage (EOC).

This will provide information about the plan's exclusions/limitations. You may be able to submit claims for services including wigs, medication prescriptions, over-the-counter medications, Health Savings Accounts plans (also known as HSA), and possibly other services. There may be tax advantages for your personal income tax for medical and/or prescription drug coverage. Talk to your accountant about this."

I'm not able to pay for my care, even with my insurance. What can I do?
Kristy Fishman: "If you have an advocate, such as a health insurance broker or plan administrator/human resources, this is a great way to ask for assistance. If you call your health insurance company for help, keep the following in mind. Insurance company employees do not make the rules. They just explain the plan's benefits, so ask them to help you. Most will be very helpful if you let them know that you need assistance. Ask a lot of questions. Ask the insurance company to explain the benefits and answer any questions you have. Ask them to give you any information concerning your questions. Ask them also to explain any plan limitations/exclusions that may apply. Ask if there is anything else you should know or be aware of. Many providers who are affiliated with large hospitals will have great sources of information. If you are currently uninsured, ask your provider about financial assistance, cash discounts, cash packages (major services), and also government programs."

What should insurance cover in terms of breast screening?
Dr. Allen Gabriel offers the following information:

- If you have a family history of breast cancer, insurance companies may provide access to early screening with mammograms and preventative treatments starting at *age thirty-five or younger.*
- If you have felt a mass in your breast, insurance companies will provide access to screening *at any age after puberty.*
- Your first mammogram for screening should be at age forty unless you fit the prior categories.

- If you have been diagnosed with dense breasts on a mammogram, insurance companies provide approval for additional diagnostic testing and referral to a specialist to discuss options for treatment.
- If you have the BRCA gene, insurance companies may provide access to preventative procedures and treatment.

I already have implants and need a mastectomy. What should I do?
In most cases, your surgeon will probably suggest that your implant is removed before mastectomy, and then do the reconstruction with a new implant after (if you desire it). Occasionally, a surgeon will do a mastectomy with the implant in place. This is then followed by a second surgery to replace the old implant with a new one. This is called implant-sparing mastectomy with a delayed implant exchange. The upside of this surgery is that you usually don't need to go through the expansion process and its risks because the implants have already created a pocket in the breast muscle. This procedure is uncommon.

I know every surgeon is different, but mine recommends reconstruction with expanders. Can you comment on this in more detail?
Dr. Allen Gabriel: "My preferred reconstructive technique *is* a two-stage expander/implant reconstruction with silicone implants, AlloDerm, and fat injection. For the first stage of reconstruction I use a tissue expander, AlloDerm, and inject Botox to paralyze the muscle so they have less pain after surgery. Once ready in about three months, I then reconstruct them with silicone implants. The highly cohesive gel implants are my preferred way, which are also known as 'gummy bear implants.' Fat injection is performed where I liposuction an area of the body, then the fat is processed and injected directly under the skin to ease with the transition of the implant and add thickness and therefore resulting in a more natural look and feel."

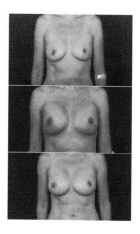

39 year old female following bilateral nipple sparing mastectomy with reconstruction with tissue expander, AlloDerm and injection of Botox into the pectoralis major muscle. In the second image, she is fully expanded prior to the placement of her final implants. The bottom image shows the same patient with the final placement of Natrelle Style 410 anatomical shaped silicone implants. By Dr. Allen Gabriel

I've read about nipple-sparing mastectomy, but what really are the advantages and disadvantages from both an oncologic and aesthetic point of view?
Dr. Allen Gabriel: "Nipple-sparing mastectomy is gaining acceptance among breast surgeons. The advantage of nipple-sparing mastectomy is the fact that the native nipple areolar complex remains on the skin, which then can be used to create an even more natural-appearing breast.

"However, there is no sensation [in the nipple], and clearly it is not functional. Some believe that if the nipple is spared, they will continue to have sensation. This is not the case.

"Candidacy can be at times complicated. First of all, there are strict oncological criteria that should be followed when offering patients nipple-sparing mastectomy. Here are the criteria that my breast surgeon and I use:

- tumor less than 3 cm
- tumors more than 3 cm from nipple
- no multicentric disease
- no triple-negative disease
- negative axillae

This is more of a conservative criteria.

"Once the patient is a candidate *oncologically*, then a plastic surgeon has to determine whether they are a *reconstructive* candidate. This is my criteria that we are planning on publishing, and I use this information to teach others:

- grade 2 ptosis (breast drooping) or better
- smaller breasts
- N: IMF <10 cm

"Basically this means, small breasts and minimal 'sagging' would make the patient a reconstructive candidate for nipple sparing. It's very common where the *breast surgeon* says, 'Yes, no problem, let's save your nipple,' and then patient see me as a *plastic surgeon* and I have to say no, and it's disappointing to them. Discuss this in detail with *both* surgeons."

What can I wear after my surgery to remain comfortable?
Elizabeth Thompson, MD, MPH, is a breast cancer previvor and founder of BFFL Co.: "Just think pure comfort. If something hurts, take it off. My suggestions for healing comfortably include the following.

1. Front-Closure Bras: Most hospitals will send you home in a nylon 1970s-style corset bra. This is unfortunate! You've just had a $20,000+ operation and need something with support, comfort, and easy access during the 'stage 1' recovery, when you still have drains.

Consider buying a bra like the Masthead Elizabeth Surgical Bra we designed, and bring it to the hospital. This brushed-backed, soft front-closure bra was designed for the operations of the current age. No Velcro against your skin, openings for the drains to exit without crimping, and no need for a fanny pack or pouch for the bulbs.

A soft bra like our Estelle Radiation Bra is not just for radiation, it's also a fantastic option for 'stage 2' healing (after your drains have been pulled).

2. Stretchy, slightly compressive undershirts. Buy a couple of these to wear over your bra before or after your drains are pulled. And many women find that they sweat when they sleep and can't tolerate anything too heavy at first. It feels good to have something snug, and I designed camisoles with exactly this in mind. Undershirts are also perfect."

3. Zip-Front Hoodies. Buy them before your surgery in cotton or cashmere, and make these a staple of your wardrobe. Everything should have pockets, as you will love to have things easily accessible. J Crew, Land's End, and Gap tend to have great hoodies all year round."

4. Vests. Vests are wonderful: breast implants or expanders can make you cold, as if you have two icepacks against your chest wall. A fleece or down vest is perfect for warmth and layering, and also hides your dressings that may make you ill-shaped and feel bulky during the first few weeks of recovery. I like ones by Patagonia and Land's End.

5. Yoga-Style Stretch Pants. Make it as easy as possible to get you pants up and down. Don't put on anything that is too tight. Many of today's yoga pants have a sleek and sophisticated look, which is a plus.

6. Flip-Flops or Clogs. Make sure to keep a few pairs of flip-flops next to the bed. Socks are impossible to pull up, and bare feet can be cold on the floor.

7. Comfort Pillow. Keep a small pillow like the Axillapilla I designed with you at all times. It will help ease the pain in your axilla after your lymph node dissection or simply decrease the friction and rubbing. This little heart-shaped pillow can be used as a neck support, seat belt protector, back pillow, or simply a tush cush."

What physical side effects may I have after breast surgery?
Lockey Maisonneuve, founder of MovingOn, an exercise program for breast cancer survivors: "If you've had breast surgery you may have these side effects:

- Rounded shoulder. After surgery, scar tissue and/or adhesions may develop across the chest wall, causing tightness and rounding of the shoulders.
- Winged scapula. After an axillary lymph node dissection, the serratus anterior may be weak, causing the shoulder blade to protrude from the body.
- Kyphosis (head tilted forward). Following a mastectomy, the tightening of the chest wall and the 'guarded' position some women will take after surgery will cause the head to lean forward, causing neck pain.
- Forward flexion. In the case of a TRAM flap procedure, it may be difficult to stand erect.
- Lordosis. In the case of a TRAM flap, curvature of the spine ('swayback') may happen due to weakened core muscles.

"All of these side effects can be managed and even corrected by starting with gentle rehabilitative exercises. Here are two of my favorite rehabilitative exercises:"

Shoulder roll: Pull shoulders up (shrug), then pull them back and drop them down.

Chest-opening stretch: Bend arms with your hands on your ears. Gently 'squeeze' your elbows apart."

I had a TRAM flap reconstruction and now have back problems. Help!
Carol Michaels, founder and creator of Recovery Fitness, an exercise program designed to help cancer patients recover from surgery and treatments: "A TRAM (transverse rectus abdominis myocutaneous) flap consists of skin, fat, rectus muscle, and blood vessels taken from the abdominal wall and transferred to the chest to reconstruct the breast. Weakness in this area can pave the way for back problems. Potential issues from TRAM flap surgery may include:

- Posture: With the diminished support from the abdominal wall, it may be difficult to stand erect, and you may develop *lordosis*, an inward curvature of the spine. You may also suffer from abdominal and lower back weakness.

- Flexibility: Upper and lower body flexibility may be compromised. You may find tightness in the hip flexors. This is due to leaning forward as a result of tightness from abdominal surgery.
- Balance: Your balance may be affected due to a decrease in core strength.
- Core strength: The rectus abdominus stabilizes the spine. Since it is no longer in the same place, other muscles have to work harder to compensate for the change.

"The first step is for you to regain range of motion—see your doctor first. A daily stretching routine for breast cancer survivors should be followed. Slowly add the pelvic tilt and bridge. Add strengthening exercises after you have achieved 80 to 90 percent of your range of motion and you are cleared by your medical professional. Remember to start easy, progress slowly, and listen to your body. It is crucial to focus on strengthening the obliques and back muscles. Because the back can be vulnerable to injury, it is necessary to learn how to lift properly.

"The following are some of the initial strength exercises that will help your recovery after a TRAM flap operation:
Exercises to Strengthen the Core

- pelvic tilt and modified Pilates exercises
- exercises to strengthen the obliques, such as the crossover crunch, modified crisscross, and the lateral crunch
- exercises to strengthen the back, such as the bridge and the bird dog
- a complete balance program should be followed; perform balance exercises such as front, side, and back leg lifts and engage in core strengthening

"There are some exercises that are contraindicated, such as sit-ups or any forceful movement to the abdominal area. If you have osteoporosis, do not perform forward bends or twists. In addition, heavy lifting should be avoided to minimize the risk of a hernia. If you have or are at risk for lymphedema, see a lymphedema specialist before beginning an exercise program. A safe exercise program will enable you to return to the activities that you enjoyed."

FREQUENTLY ASKED QUESTIONS ABOUT NIPPLE RECONSTRUCTION AND TATTOOING

I had reconstruction with implants. Now the skin on my reconstructed nipple feels so thin and fragile. Can still get a tattoo?
Dr. Ariel N. Rad: "Yes. Tattoo ink is placed in the dermis, the thickest part of the skin. If you have had implant reconstruction, there is a layer of fat between the dermis and the implant no matter how thin the tissue layer is (unless the implant has caused excessive stretching of the skin). When done properly, the ink doesn't penetrate below this tissue layer, so it is exceedingly rare, if not impossible, to harm the implant. Seek the skill of a *licensed professional* tattoo artist."

How soon after reconstruction can I get an areola tattoo? Do I need permission or clearance from my surgeon to have an areola tattoo done?
Areola Architect Cathi Locati is highly sought after by New York area plastic surgeons and treatment centers for her realistic nipple and areola tattoos. She explains: "All open wounds and scabs in the areola area must be gone and healed before considering tattooing. Fresh or currently healing stitches, wounds, and scabs are OK as long as they are outside of the areola area. It is really a case by case basis. We contact your surgeon and double-check with him or her about timing if it seems to be an issue and you want the tattoo sooner."

I'm concerned about the cost of nipple and areola tattooing, which I have heard can be up to $2,500.
Currently, according to the Women's Health and Cancer Rights Act of 1998, "patients whose health plan covers mastectomies are entitled to full

insurance coverage for postmastectomy reconstruction, including nipple micropigmentation." Your tattoo artist should write her invoice so that you can submit it to your insurance company and be covered. Speak with your insurance company about how this should be done.

My plastic surgeon is urging me to have him/her do my tattoo. How do the nipples and areolas an artist creates differ from other tattoo artist and surgeons/ nurses tattoo work?

Cathi Locati: "You are not bound by any insurance company to choose a surgeon over a tattoo artist. Other tattoo artists' and surgeons' or nurses' tattoo work can appear standard. They use a small needle to 'fill in' the [areola] circle and 'color-added' discs similar to a pink coin using one design for both the right and the left side. Photorealism, 3-D areolas and nipples by a highly trained and specialized areola architect appear similar to fine artwork done by the Old Masters such as Michelangelo, DaVinci, etc. We create a distinct right areola that looks round and protruding, and a distinctly different left areola—not just two flat pink coins.

"Custom-created artwork by areola architects is virtually indistinguishable from the actual body part we are replicating. The final outcome when choosing an areola architect verses a regular tattoo artist or surgeon/ nurse, who are trained medical providers but not trained fine artists, is dramatically different. For example, I mark arrows on my patients' chests dropping down from the supra-sternal fossa (base of neck in front below the esophagus, tracheotomy area) in both directions to remind myself as I am tattooing, where the light is coming from and where the shadows would fall. This artistic technique gives the most natural result. The best test? Compare before and after of your surgeon's work and an artist's photos side by side. The choice is usually quite clear."

What should I be looking for in terms of before and after photos?

Cathi Locati: "The type and scope of artistic skill through photos that an artist or surgeon is willing to show you is going to be the best indicator of how their areolas and nipples will look when created with a tattoo machine.

"Or ask them to take the sixty-second test, which asks them to draw their rendition of their best areola and nipple using a regular ballpoint pen on paper. Remember, the pen point of a regular pen is usually wider than the needles they use to implant pigments in a tattoo. If they can't do it well with a pen…this is how they are going to tattoo with a machine and ink!"

What is "touching up" a tattoo?

Dr. Laura Reed explains: "There are two types of touch-ups: Any first-time (new) cosmetic or medical tattoo must be considered a two-part process (sometimes more) for optimal results. The reason is that it is a tattoo on a human canvas. If an area bleeds or exudes lymph, it may not 'hold' the pigment well. That area may heal lighter and not match the rest of the tattoo. So a touch-up is essentially another procedure that provides the opportunity for the artist to adjust those areas. Color, size, and shape can also be adjusted at this touch-up procedure, which more accurately would be called a 'refinement' visit.

"The other type of touch-up can be described more accurately as a 'refresher' or 'maintenance' procedure. Over time, the tattoo pigments will fade, and a procedure to refresh the colors must be performed. Areola tattoos can typically go longer without needing a color refresher because they are covered up by clothing. They are not exposed to damaging UV light on a daily basis like permanent makeup on the face is. The need for a refresher is subjective and can be determined by the patient. On average, maintenance will be necessary every three to five years. It is essentially a re-tattooing, but the procedure is shorter because the design and placement is already done."

Can you provide a detailed aftercare program?

Dr. Laura Reed: "Although aftercare regimens can vary among cosmetic tattoo practitioners, this is my protocol.

"Immediately after a procedure, I bandage my patient. First I apply a double antibiotic ointment on top of the tattoos followed by a sterile, latex-free, nonstick gauze pad (Telfa is a common brand name) secured by hypoallergenic tape. To ensure minimum loss of color and scab formation, I tell her not to cleanse the area with anything (even water) for six to twelve hours. She will continue to apply ointments and wear pads for the first week of healing (approximately seven days, up to ten days).

"For the first several days, the woman should change her nonstick pad several times per day (absolute minimum of twice per day). She should apply a topical antibiotic ointment with a clean cotton swab (fingertips are not advised due to potential bacteria). The antibiotic can be purchased over the counter. If a woman has previously used a triple antibiotic ointment (brand name Neosporin) with no allergic reaction, she may use that. However, many people are allergic to the neomycin component of that ointment. Therefore, if she is uncertain, it is preferred she use what most dermatologists recommend—a double antibiotic ointment (brand name Polysporin). It contains the same antibiotic components as the triple ointment minus the neomycin.

"After using the antibiotic ointment for three or four days, the woman can then switch to using clean Vaseline or Aquaphor ointment for the remainder of the week. The purpose of using ointments is to minimize the chance of infection and prevent the tattoos from drying out. Keeping them moist will also help prevent scabbing and itching, thereby improving comfort. Note: On rare occasions, a contact dermatitis may develop from using too much ointment. When that occurs, itching may increase along with what appears to be a rash. If that happens, the woman should stop using the products and contact her tattooist right away. Typically that resolves by keeping the tattoo dry or applying some hydrocortisone cream.

"During healing, it helps if the woman can go topless/braless as much as possible. She should apply her ointment as usual but leave the pad off, allowing oxygen to aid the healing process. However, when she must wear clothing and is in bed, she should wear her nonstick pads for protection. If she is a "stomach sleeper," she should also sleep on her side or back during her recovery week. The areola tattoo(s) should always be protected and not rubbed, scratched, or irritated in any way.

"Baths and showers are permitted if the tattoos are not exposed to a direct, hard shower spray. During the first healing week, she should apply a thicker coat of ointment before showering or bathing to repel any soap and water. Soaking in a bathtub or hot tub or taking a long, hot, steamy shower or sauna should be avoided completely for two weeks. Also swimming in an ocean, lake, river, or pool should be avoided for two weeks. During the second week of healing, a mild cleanser can be used to lightly wash the tattoos with clean fingertips (for example, Cetaphil, Neutrogena, Ivory, baby wash, etc.) and gently rinsed.

"Once the main healing is complete, there may still be some mild peeling or flaking of skin. The woman can then apply body or moisture lotion. However, she should not use any 'antiaging' lotions or cosmetics on her tattoo(s) that contain bleaching or exfoliating agents (for example, AHAs)—they can cause additional peeling and fading of the pigments."

What are some things that will affect the color of my tattoo?
Dr. Laura Reed: "All tattoos fade over time. However, the longevity of nipple-areola tattoos is usually greater since they are protected from the sun—UV exposure is the main culprit in fading tattoos and permanent makeup. After the follow-up procedure, the tattoo should last several years before needing a color refresher. Factors affecting fading include general health, UV exposure (sun or tanning beds), smoking, metabolism, and medications."

This sounds odd, but I heard that an MRI can affect the color of my tattoo.
Dr. Laura Reed: "There is some confusion about cosmetic tattooing and MRI procedures. It is safe for a woman with an areola tattoo to have an MRI performed. However, she should notify her radiologist and the MRI technician that she has the tattoo and that it was created with pigments containing iron oxides. Laser treatments on or near the tattoo should be avoided since the laser can change the color of the pigments. If the treatment is necessary, the physician and laser technician should be informed so they can shield the tattoo as much as possible."

Will I be able to donate blood—either to the Red Cross or to a family member, if needed—after my tattoo? I would hate to think that I can't!
Dr. Laura Reed: "Under current Red Cross blood donor eligibility guidelines, the woman may be able to donate without waiting a year if she had her

tattoo performed *under the supervision of a physician* or in a facility inspected by (regulated by) the health department. State laws vary and will need to be investigated, and she can discuss that with the health historian who performs the screening."

I had a mastectomy and chose not to have either reconstruction or nipple tattoos. What are my other options for nonsurgical reconstruction or ornamentation?
Cathi Locati: "You can absolutely tattoo anything you want. Dragonflies, flowers, illusion undergarments (bras, vests, seashells, lace, corsets, etc). You're only limited by your imagination. Run wild. Through great ongoing communication with your artist, we work toward your ultimate beauty ideas.

"I have also invented a revolutionary new tattoo technique, 7th Dimension Illusion Breastmounds, to 'paint' two photorealistic, full breasts onto the flat chest barrel, creating the illusion of round, soft, protruding, pointed breasts complete with areolas and nipples using permanent organic ink. The name 7th Dimension comes from the magical illusion that tricks the eye into believing its seeing the real thing; when the patient turns to the side, the illusion holds. Think of it as nonsurgical reconstruction! The viewer knows the chest is flat and that the breasts aren't really there, but the eye sees protruding breasts as though they were actual weighted breasts." For more information, see www.cathilocatico.com.

QUESTIONS TO ASK YOUR BREAST SURGEON
Experience
Are you board-certified in plastic and reconstructive surgery? Is your certification up to date?

How many breast reconstruction procedures have you done?

How will you work or coordinate with my breast surgeon?

How will my surgeries be coordinated with other treatments (chemotherapy, radiation, etc.)?

May I see before and after pictures of reconstruction?

Can you put me in touch with some of your past patients?

Types of Reconstruction

Based on the stage and location of my tumor and medical history, what are my options for reconstruction?

Please explain the difference between autologous (flap) reconstruction and implant reconstruction.

How long can I wait to have reconstruction if I haven't decided yet? How long do I have to wait between procedures?

Which procedure gives the most natural results?

Will I have scars, and where will they be?

What are the risks associated with each type of reconstruction?

How many procedures will I need for each type of reconstruction from start to finish?

I may want to reconstruct only my affected breast: what do you do to achieve symmetry? Do you suggest bilateral mastectomy and reconstruction?

Can I change the size of my breasts through reconstruction?

What will my breasts feel like after each procedure?

Will I have sensation in the reconstructed breast?

Please explain the different nipple and areola reconstruction techniques?

What nipple reconstruction procedure guarantees better results?

Could the reconstructed nipple flatten?

What is the time of healing and pain level for each procedure?

Can nipple reconstruction cause health issues?

Surgical Procedures

How long does each surgery take?

Where will my incisions be?

What type of anesthesia is used? What are the associated risks?

How are complications handled?

Will I need drains?

Will I need a blood transfusion? Can I donate my own blood?

What is the post-op process?

Will I need to do anything special to prepare for surgery?

Should I stop taking certain medications before procedures?

How long after each procedure before I can resume my medication?

Do I need to let my oncology team know about the different procedures I am about to undergo?

What is the length of the hospital stay for each procedure?

What can I expect in terms of pain and pain management?

Recovery at Home

Realistically, how long will it take me to recover from a particular procedure?

Will I have to do anything to care for my incisions/scars during recovery?

How do I care for drains and when will they be removed?

What are warning signs for infection and other complications?

What if I get arm swelling?

How do I manage pain?

Do I need to do anything to prepare my house?

What medical supplies will I need to buy?

Will I need any special food or drinks?

Will I need extra help at home? Can I get a professional nurse to visit me at my home?

Will I be able to shower and bathe? When?

When can I resume normal activity and driving?

What kind of exercise can I do and when can I start?

Will I need physical therapy?

When can I go back to work?

Aesthetic Outcome

What are my options if I'm not happy with the results?

How long will I have to wait to get revision surgeries, if needed?

My Future Health

Will having reconstruction interfere with mammograms in the future?

Reconstructed breast feel different than natural breasts; who should do my future breast exams?

What happens if my cancer comes back?

What happens if my breast implants rupture or leak?

BREAST RECONSTRUCTION AND NIPPLE TATTOOING TIPS FROM SURVIVORS

"The best thing you can do for yourself is research your diagnosis, the procedures, medications, and treatments, as well as options that may be available to you. Because I informed myself and initiated discussions with my doctors, based on the type and location of my tumor I was able to have a skin-saving/nipple-saving mastectomy. I would have lost mine if I hadn't spoken up. Having the exterior of my breast intact was a huge psychological advantage for me in my healing process. I want other women going through the process to know that as hard as it is to deal with breast cancer in particular, you need to actively participate in the treatment and recovery process to make it truly successful for yourself." —Dawn Gum

"Postsurgery: take it easy, don't push yourself, rest, get enough sleep, don't resist medication, stay in front of the pain. Accept help from others. Allow people to bring you meals, help with your children (provide rides for you and your children), have others run your errands. Friends don't know what to do and want to do something, so let them, even if you think it is silly. Graciously accept gifts. Realize you are going to disappoint others, you may say you will do something and then you can't do it because you don't feel well." —Iris Lee Knell

"Use a blog or online journal to update others on your status. It helps with fatigue and needing to repeat yourself over and over." —Iris Lee Knell, L.C.S.W., founder of Chemocessories (www.chemocessories.org)

"If postsurgery you ever feel down, remember it is not so unusual because breast cancer has a huge emotional component. Talk to someone. Do *not* bottle that up. Most major hospital systems have some sort of therapist that breast cancer gals can talk to before and after surgery." —Carla Joy Zambelli, www.ihavebreastcancerblog.me

"As soon as I got the OK to shower, I took one every morning and thoroughly enjoyed every delicious drop of water! And here was the big one for me…I did not spend my day in bed! I felt so much better in the recliner or on the couch. To get up, shower, get dressed, and sit at the table for breakfast was so therapeutic for me; besides it forced me to walk around and get a bit of exercise." —Sherry Stose, RN

"The best advice I can give is to follow your doctors' instructions, and ask questions if you don't know the answer or are confused. Also *rest*. If I was doing it all over again I would've rested more. I did not do enough of that." —Carla Joy Zambelli

"When you asked how I chose implant over tissue, it really didn't take long. In our first consultation my plastic surgeon said that the tissue option produced less optimal cosmetic results and you'd come out looking like a football. But by that point I was already leaning toward implants because I didn't want additional surgeries if I could help it… I feel like less is more where surgery is concerned." —Jackie Fox, author of *From Zero to Mastectomy*

"Tip to Minimize nipple deflation during healing. Buy a Dr. Scholl's Corn and Callus Remover. Discard any liquid that comes with it. Cut in half and press two halves together. Place two halves around a reconstructed nipple before wearing a bra. The corn remover protects the nipple and does not allow it to be flattened." - Lana Koifman

"I try to share with all survivors the importance of physical therapy. It helps so much with scar tissue and cuts down the risk of lymphedema. It has allowed me to have great range of motion. I feel PT is vital to all survivors." —Gaye Moore-Lewis

"Move your body. You might not be able to work out like you used to but just do it. Nothing lifts your life force like getting the blood pumping and your chi flowing! Look for a restorative yoga or tai chi class. Find a local indoor pool where you can do a few leisurely laps. The endorphins will lift your spirits, and a good mood = soul food. Your body is responding to the signals you send it so make them as healthy as possible. When I was in treatment, I approached the flat-grade treadmill like it was Mt. Etna. But, I made it ten minutes and felt like an Olympic athlete and the end!" —Jennifer Alhasa, cancer coach

"I kind of liked my new 'friend' that balanced out my front! They did amazing things to accomplish a single reconstruction, as implants were not an option. I got a tummy tuck, new belly button (these were not extra but needed, as it was part of the process), symmetry lift for my other breast to match, used liposuction to fill a huge hole that showed above my blouses from where they dug the tumor out, and fixed a hideous two-inch round scar from wound care near a radiated spot. There are countless possibilities of what surgeons can do, but it will take some time." —Lynn Jones

CHAPTER FOUR

SCAR TREATMENT

YOU MAY END UP WITH SCARS as part of your cancer treatment. A scar is your body's response to an injury, and is part of the natural healing process. It is composed of a layer of fibrous tissue that replaces your original skin and its function. Fortunately, there are sophisticated techniques to minimize the look of your scars, from over-the-counter topical treatments to complex surgeries for significant scars.

If you want to treat scars, it is important to do it *immediately*, states dermatologist Dr. Jeanine Downie: "It sounds counterintuitive, and most people assume a scar should heal completely before any cosmetic treatment, but the newer and fresher the scar, the easier it is to manipulate and fix. Plus you may end up needing to have more treatments, and therefore spend more money if you wait."

Here are some commonly used treatments for four different types of scars: flat (level with skin surface), raised (keloids and hypertrophic), depressed (sunken or concave), and contractures (from extreme injury like burns, sometimes caused by significant radiation burn).

FLAT SCARS
Topical Treatments
These may include the following:
- A prescription cream like Biafine (particularly good for radiation scars.)

Scars can be made much worse by sun exposure! It is very important to use appropriate sun protection on scars daily, as inadequate protection can lead to permanent darkening.

- Over-the-counter topical treatments include ScarAway Silicone Gel Sheets (see below), Bio Oil, Mederma Advanced Scar Gel, Cimeosil Scar Gel, or Radiaplex Rx Wound Gel Dressing. Dr. Downie adds: "Make sure whatever treatment you choose to use a gentle cleanser on the area. Good drugstore brands include Dove, Cetaphil, and Aveeno."
- Natural treatments such as cocoa butter and vitamin E oil.
- Topical silicone gel and silicone sheeting: Silicone gel sheeting may help reduce the appearance of old scars. It can also inhibit the formation of new scars because it increases hydration to the skin, protects the skin from bacteria and possible infection, and can reduce discomfort while a scar heals. Silicone sheeting seems to work very well, and it is inexpensive and readily available.

Lasers

Many lasers used for cosmetic purposes can do wonders on scarring too. For permanent dark spots, broken blood vessels, or skin that looks more sun-damaged than before treatment, the Excel V laser may be used. The Fraxel Re: Store laser may be used for radiation burn.

Compression

Pressure taping a scar postsurgery appears to work well, particularly for burns. This technique removes tension away from the edges of the scar so it heals more uniformly and more quickly.

Scar Camouflage

Sometimes it is enough to just lighten the look of a scar so it blends in with your skin. A professional tattoo artist can help by adding skin-toned pigments into the area and blend them into the surrounding skin. As with nipple tattooing, find an artist experienced in this technique. Please see our section on nipple tattooing for more information.

RAISED SCARS

There are basically two kinds of raised scars: keloids and hypertrophic (or hyperplastic).

- Keloids are long, darkened raised scars that go beyond the boundaries of the original incision or injury. They continue to grow long after the initial healing is complete, sometimes for up to two years, and can be itchy and irritated. Keloids are often the result of skin that creates too much scar tissue after injury and does not flatten over time. They can be a simple cosmetic concern or sometimes more serious, even hampering movement.

- Hypertrophic scars look like keloids, but do not extend beyond the original boundaries of the incision or injury. They also do not continue to grow after the initial healing period and will eventually flatten and fade.

It is important for your doctor to identify whether your scar is keloid or hypertrophic before treating it because these scars react differently to treatment.

Steroid Injections

Your doctor may recommend a kenalog injection, in which a diluted steroid like cortisone is injected directly into the scar. Steroids are powerful anti-inflammatories and can help soften and shrink the scar. However, you will still be left with a scar even though it is now flatter and smaller. Sometimes dermatologists combine the injections with scar bandages, massage, and laser treatments to resurface the skin and reduce the look of the scar.

> **NEW HELP FOR KELOID SCARS.**
> *"A new take on an old therapy is now showing great promise—radiation. This can be very intimidating to the cancer patient, who may have undergone radiation as a part of their treatment. However, we have superficial radiotherapy (SRT) that can treat keloids very effectively. SRT does not come with the side effects of other types of radiation, such as inflammation of the skin and skin breakdown. The results are pretty impressive."*
> —Dr. Shannon Campbell

Topical Silicone Gel and Silicone Sheeting

See above.

Massage

To encourage scar fading and flattening, you might be urged to try "cross-fiber" or transfriction massage. Use one or two fingers to gently press and massage your scar perpendicular to the line of the scar. This helps remodel the scar and ensures that the collagen fibers of the scar are aligned properly. At first your scar may appear redder, but as time goes on it will fade noticeably. You can follow the massage with vitamin E oil. Ask your doctors for more massage techniques.

Vascular Laser

Some dermatologists recommend the 1540 laser IPL Intense Pulsed Light treatments to reduce redness, followed by the 1540 Non ablative fractional Erbium Laser to flatten a raised scar. Other lasers used include pulsed dye laser treatments like the Vbeam.

Scar Revision

Scar revision means surgically removing the old scar and "replacing" it with a new, more discreet one. Dr. Debra Jaliman notes: "Some people after surgery have very good healing and minimal scarring with good wound care. Others do get keloids. If the keloids don't respond to [other] treatment they can be numbed with a local anesthetic and cut out. Then the skin is restitched and good wound care performed. The outcome should be better."

One scar revision technique is called Z-plasty. This procedure literally makes a zigzag pattern of incisions into the scar. This works to elongate a contracted (puckered) scar like a burn, or realign the scar line so it is less visible.

Your surgeon may also include tissue substitutes or tissue expansion in his or her scar revision procedure if there is not enough healthy tissue to adequately cover the scar.

Please note: some types of skin are predisposed to creating keloid or hypertrophic scars. In this case, scar revision surgery may not work because the body will simply create another raised scar when the old one is removed. Speak to your dermatologist beforehand to avoid a costly, unsuccessful procedure.

DEPRESSED SCARS

Depressed scars are also referred to as sunken or concave scars and appear as divots in the flesh. They can be as minor as acne scars or as significant as major denting and volume loss in a large area such as after a lumpectomy. In this case, additional surgery may be needed.

Fat Grafting (Autologous Fat Transfer)

Fat grafting may be appropriate for acne scars, radiation burns, and scarring, or a moderate sunken scar from lumpectomy or other surgery. Fat grafting uses fat taken from another area of the body—usually the abdomen or hips—to create a web of support under the area and thus raise it. It can also smooth irregular contours such as retracted scars from breast reconstruction or liposuction.

Fillers (Percutaneous Scar Release)

Sometimes collagen or other fillers may be used to plump up shallow sunken scars. These can be particularly helpful for acne scars, but as with any application of fillers, they are not a permanent solution. See our section on fillers above.

Subcision

This is minor surgical technique may be used in conjunction with fillers to help with a light to moderate scar. Your doctor will use a needle to cut a tunnel under the scar that can heal on its own with the body's collagen or be filled with a hyaluronic acid filler.

CONTRACTURES

Contractures are scars in which the skin is pulled together after an injury, and they can appear when a significant amount of skin has been lost, as in the case of a burn. These scars tighten the skin and can restrict movement.

Silicone Sheeting

See above.

Skin Grafting

Skin grafting includes the transplantation of skin from one area of the body to another. A common type is the removal of a thin layer of healthy skin from a donor site, called a split-thickness graft. The layer of skin is processed through a mesh made of flexible material that allows it to expand (although it can also lead to a pebbled appearance). This method is used to cover large areas of affected tissue.

Two other graft techniques are full-thickness graft, in which the entire thickness of the skin of the donor site is cut away and grafted, and composite graft, which excises skin and underlying cartilage or other tissue.

Laser treatments are sometimes used after skin grafting to create a more uniform skin texture and tone. Skin grafting is a complex procedure that requires special skill to achieve a good cosmetic outcome; please speak with your doctor in detail.

Tissue Expansion

In this technique, an inflatable balloon is placed under the skin and expanded through saline injections over time to stretch the skin. Once the skin has been stretched adequately, the expander and scar are removed. The stretched skin is then used to replace the original scar issue. Z-plasty and flap repair are also sometimes employed.

Z-plasty

See above.

CHAPTER FIVE

DENTAL CARE DURING CANCER TREATMENT

CANCER TREATMENT DOES NOT ALWAYS CAUSE dental issues, but therapies like chemo and/or targeted radiation can have unpleasant and uncomfortable side effects such as inflamed gums, teeth stains, pain, tooth decay, or even tooth loss that can affect self-esteem and interrupt healing. Fortunately there are ways to avoid these issues.

Practicing good oral health is important at every stage of life, but before and during cancer treatment it is absolutely critical. Problems often happen because a person's mouth is not healthy before radiation starts, so be sure to see your dentist before starting treatment.

This chapter will cover:

- Dental care before your treatment
- Chemotherapy, radiation, and dental health
- Dental care during treatment: brushing and cleaning, nutrition
- Solutions for commonly found mouth and dental issues during cancer treatment

We want to reassure you that many dental and mouth problems from cancer treatment are temporary and there *are* solutions for short- and long-term effects to help you look and feel your best during and after your treatment.

MANAGING THE COST OF DENTAL CARE.

Dental care is expensive and an increasing issue for many people. Lack of dental insurance (or in some cases, inadequate insurance), job loss, fear, and other factors can cause people to put oral health on the back burner. These issues can be compounded if you are uncertain about how your financial life will be affected. For instance, will you be able to continue working and maintain medical insurance? Will your treatment impact your family member's jobs?

Proactive oral health care before starting cancer treatment is absolutely critical: there are excellent options to receive quality dental care while minimizing costs:

- *Check out your local dental school. Some have teaching clinics that offer services by students closely monitored by experienced professors. One such school is New York University in Manhattan, which offers excellent services for very little cost.*
- *Schools for dental hygienists can also offer services that allow students to gain experience with experienced dentists overseeing the procedures.*
- *The Bureau of Primary Health Care, a service of the Health Resources and Services Administration, lists community health centers across the country that offer free or reduced-cost dental care. They can be reached on the web at www.bphc.hrsa.gov, or by calling 888-275-4772.*
- *The Center for Medicaid also sponsors programs for people qualifying for Medicaid, Medicare, or Children's Health Program,*
- *Finally, certain charities, such as the United Way, may help assist you in finding low- or no-cost dental care.*

HOW CHEMOTHERAPY AND RADIATION AFFECT THE MOUTH

Like skin and hair, your mouth is affected by chemotherapy and radiation treatments. Dr. Alina Krivitsky explains: "Chemotherapeutic agents can affect rapidly dividing cells of the target tumor, oral epithelium lining, and vascular, inflammatory, and healing response of the oral cavity. These changes may cause mucositis [mouth sores], secondary infections, and painful food consumption. Chemotherapeutic agents also target bone marrow cells, increasing the risk of infection." The latter can be especially dangerous when blood counts are low.

Of course, not all chemo drugs may cause problems. Speak to your oncology team, and see our FAQ at the end of the chapter.

Radiation

Unlike chemotherapy, radiation tends to produce more long-term oral complications. Radiation can alter bone that is in the pathway of the radiation beam, notes Dr. Steven Bornfeld: "This means that any injury to the mouth in the irradiated areas will heal more slowly—in fact may not heal at all."

Head and neck radiation treatments are more likely to cause oral complications, most notably dry mouth and mouth sores. Some may be short term and end at the conclusion of treatment, while others are long term and can be permanent, such as dry mouth, being prone to cavities, and bone loss due to the reduction of blood to the jawbone during treatment. The side effects of radiation depend on the location of the beam and high-dose per fraction rate; in other words, the effects are local to the area where you receive the radiation. This puts the patient at a *lifetime* risk of osteoradionecrosis of the jaw, known as ONJ (see below). The risk for ONJ is in direct proportion to the amount of radiation the patient receives. Since long-term implications for dental health are more prevalent, giving extra attention to dental help is of the utmost importance—see more below.

PREPARING YOUR MOUTH FOR CANCER TREATMENT

Get a clean bill of dental health before starting cancer treatment to avoid the need for any invasive dental procedures during it. Cancer patients face a higher risk of infection due to a depressed immune system, and they can heal more slowly. Getting ready for treatment means paying attention to the little things that may previously have been monitored but not dealt with. Your dentist should work closely with your oncology team to bring your mouth to optimal health.

Have a thorough dental evaluation, including the following:

- A full dental cleaning including scaling (scraping tartar)
- Full set of x-rays
- Complete tooth prognosis (checking tooth health)

- Full periodontal prognosis (checking health of the gums)
- Complete check of dental implants, dentures, bridges, and other prostheses that can rub and irritate the mouth lining and gums (and increase risk of infection)
- A fluoride treatment to reduce chance of cavities

You and your dentist may also decide to do the following:

- Extract any "unsalvageable" teeth and fill severe cavities. Do this *well in advance* of chemotherapy or radiation so you have enough time to heal thoroughly.
- Complete any significant dental work, such as root canals—allowing at least three weeks of recovery before cancer treatment starts
- Remove braces, particularly on children and adolescents
- Stop smoking
- Dr. Gregg Schneider suggests you start taking L-glutamine to help prevent dry mouth, as well as a probiotic like lactobacillus sporogenes, which may help mouth sores. These can be found at health food stores and some pharmacies.

ORAL CARE DURING CANCER TREATMENT
Brushing and Cleaning Measures

Whether you encounter mouth issues or not, continue your previous, *thorough* oral care regimen during your treatment, but make some simple changes:

- Brush with an extra soft toothbrush at least twice a day. Try rinsing your toothbrush in hot water before brushing to soften it thoroughly.
- Avoid "whitening" toothpastes, which can contain mild abrasives
- Check with your dental team to see if you should be placed on high-fluoride toothpaste
- Avoid mouthwashes that are flavored and/or contain alcohol

- Floss daily—but *only* if advised to do so. Renita Sansom, a dental hygienist with Dental Oncology Professionals North Texas, suggests you speak to your dentist before flossing. He or she might consider your history of illness, blood count, and other indicators of health before allowing you to floss. If you are able to floss, she recommends waxed tape or floss only.
- If you have dental implants, bridges, dentures, or removable appliances, check with your doctor to see if they require special cleaning.
- Rinse mouth frequently to remove bacteria, lubricate tissue, and soothe sore gums. Gargling and rinsing the mouth with salt water without swallowing is the cheapest, easiest remedy to keep your mouth clean.
- Drink more water.
- Examine your mouth daily to monitor any changes! A good lighted mirror can help.
- If you cannot tolerate flossing and brushing your teeth daily, or are not getting proper nutrition due to inflammation in your mouth, speak to your medical team about pain management.
- Prepare to see your dentist every three months.
- Avoid invasive dental work if at all possible.

Supportive Nutritional Measures

Help your body heal by incorporating a few dietary changes, courtesy of Drs. Magali Chohan and Gregg Schneider.

- Adhere to a healthy diet with lots of fruits and vegetables, such as a balanced Mediterranean diet with no high fructose corn syrup or hydrogenated fats.
- Cook with olive oil and use herbs and spices like garlic, turmeric, rosemary, and thyme. However, avoid pungent spices like chili, pepper, cinnamon, nutmeg, and mustard.

- Avoid excessive sugar: we all know that refined sugar causes cavities, which is something you definitely don't want during treatment, but sugar also fills you up and can lead to a less nutrient-rich diet. Your body needs adequate nutrition to help it heal during this time more than ever.

- Eat small regular meals and cook with high-quality fresh ingredients whenever possible.

- Increase your protein intake.

- Drink green and white tea: In addition to being a potent antioxidant, according to overwhelming scientific evidence, green tea can aid in dental health. Many nutritionists advise drinking tea every day, but always check with the professionals on your medical team, as they may ask you to limit your intake during chemotherapy.

> **Emergency dental work.**
> *The best thing to do is avoid having to have dental work during cancer treatment by prepping your mouth well and dealing with any issues before treatment starts. According to Dr. Alina Krivitsky: "If emergency treatment is necessary, it is usually recommended to base treatment on the patient's current white blood cell count (ability to fight infection). However, in most cases, palliative treatment is recommended with antibiotics taken a couple of days prior to treatment to minimize bacterial count and chance of infection spread. If treatment is absolutely necessary, then it is recommended to do it in between chemotherapy/radiation sessions... Judgment is always based on individual basis and blood counts." Your dentist should work closely with your oncology team to determine the best and safest time in your treatment cycle to have the work done.*

- Avoid foods that are spicy, salty, or require extra chewing.
- You can also start a vitamin regimen. Check with your team, but this might include:
  - a high-quality multivitamin and mineral supplement
  - Extra vitamin D3 supplements
  - omega-3 fish oil (be sure to check with your doctor, especially if you are taking blood thinners)
  - L-glutamine and probiotics

ORAL SIDE EFFECTS OF CANCER TREATMENTS

Here are the most commonly reported side effects:

1. Mucositis or Mouth Sores

Usually simply referred to as "mouth sores," mucositis is a generalized inflammation of the mouth with accompanying painful, swollen sores. It affects the entire lining of the mouth and digestive tract in conjunction with decreased saliva production. It is the most commonly experienced side effects of both chemotherapy and radiation.

Most cancer patients—particularly those being treated with both radiation and chemotherapy—will face annoying and sometimes debilitating mouth sores that can, in some cases, leave the entire soft palate of the mouth raw and extremely painful. Preexisting conditions may worsen mouth sores too. These include diabetes, kidney disease, HIV/AIDS, alcohol use, poor oral hygiene, and previous cancer treatments.

Symptoms to look for include:

- Swollen and red mouth and gums
- Whitish sores in mouth (resembling canker sores)
- Difficulty chewing, talking, and swallowing
- Pain during eating
- Thickened saliva and/or mucus

Mucositis can be dangerous because it makes dental care (and sometimes even eating) painful and may cause you to avoid good oral hygiene. However, try to stick with good habits, as mouth sores can create entry points for bacteria and viruses and invite harmful infection. Pain management is a *must* not only for comfort but so mouth sores don't cause delays in or even terminate your treatment. If sores worsen to the point that you do not want to eat, particularly if you are already experiencing nausea from your treatment, a liquid diet or eventual hospitalization can occur, greatly increasing the chance of secondary issues such as malnutrition and a further decrease in immunity.

Mouth sores generally start within one to two weeks of treatment and can last anywhere from one to six weeks. The good thing, however, is that they generally disappear when your treatment is over!

Solutions for Mouth Sores

Below are some general solutions, but please refer to our chart for more comprehensive suggestions in our Appendix.

Magic Mouthwashes (Pink Mouthwashes)

Magic Mouthwashes are compounded mouth rinses and favorites of dentists who treat cancer patients. They soothe the mouth, reduce pain and inflammation, reduce the risk of infection, and calm sour stomach that may occur during treatment.

Although dentists will mix their mouthwashes differently, they generally consist of a steroid, an antibiotic, an antihistamine, an antifungal, and an antacid. They may not be as complicated as you might think; one of our experts has her pharmacy mix a combination of lidocaine (to numb the mouth), Benadryl (the antihistamine that gives the mouthwash its "pinkness"), nystatin (prescription antifungal), and Maalox (for sour stomach that can accompany the sores). You can also make your own using over-the-counter medications like these. Just check with your dentist first.

Change Your Dental Care Routine

Sometimes just changing your dental care routine can help:

- Use foam toothbrushes, and if sores are really bad, brush every four hours to promote moisturization and decrease the possibility of infections.
- Keep lips moisturized with a lip balm (see Skin Chapter for suggestions)
- Avoid smoking or chewing tobacco.
- Avoid aspirin or nonsteroidal anti-inflammatory pain relievers like Motrin or Naprosyn (which may increase the risk of bleeding).

Nutrition

You can help mouth sores with changes in your eating habits:

- Avoid hot/spicy foods; sour foods like pickles; and acidic foods, including condiments like horseradish, mustard, and vinegar. Tomato-based condiments can be irritating too.
- Avoid acidic fruit like oranges, grapefruit, and kiwi, and even tomatoes. Instead, eat nonacidic fruits like bananas, melons, and watermelon. These can be great frozen too.
- Eat a soft, bland diet if mouth sores are bad, and, if necessary, go for liquids and purees like vegetable soups and vegetable or fruit purees. Try yogurt, well-cooked rice, and pasta.
- Eat popsicles, frozen yogurt, or other chilled items.
- Avoid crunchy food, which can damage the mouth: crackers, chips, pretzels, breadsticks, granola/muesli, crispy fried foods, etc.
- Try oatmeal: oatmeal is rich in mucilage, a natural lubricant, and can help with dry mouth. Be sure to cook is very well.
- Avoid acidic drinks such as orange juice, and instead drink nonacidic beverages like apple juice, water (best!), and nonsugary sports drinks.
- Avoid fizzy drinks if they bother you: if you like soda, you can let it stand for a while to reduce the carbonation or stir vigorously before drinking.
- Use a straw.
- Avoid, or at least limit, coffee and caffeine. You might try tea instead.

CRYOTHERAPY FOR MOUTH SORES?

Cryotherapy is a fancy term for sucking on ice chips or cubes. The coldness of the ice decreases the blood flow to the mouth and can reduce the mouth's exposure to chemotherapy drugs. In fact, this simple way of cooling and coating your mouth may prevent mouth sores. In addition to sucking on ice chips during the day, consider using them about five minutes before your chemotherapy/radiation and during the first thirty minutes, according to a 2009 article in Journal of Implant & Advanced Clinical Dentistry.

2. Dry Mouth (Xerostomia)

Dry mouth is caused by the change in the secretory cells of the salivary glands which in turn decreases the production of saliva. Radiation, in particular, can lead to dry mouth. In addition to being painful and making it difficult to eat (and thus compromising nutrition), dry mouth can also lead to tooth decay because the mouth does not produce enough of the moisturizing, cleansing, and acid-buffering abilities of saliva, explains Dr. Michael Sinkin. It can also cause difficulty speaking and swallowing (dysphagia).

With chemotherapy, dry mouth can begin as little as one week after your treatment starts and peaks about two weeks later. With radiation, the severity of dry mouth depends on the level of radiation, and usually begins between two to three weeks after initial treatment. It can last six to eight weeks, so be sure to arm yourself with some treatments in Appendix. In general:

- Suck on ice chips, and try sugarless lemon drops or mint.
- Try a toothpaste for sensitive teeth (ask your dentist).
- Use moisturizing mouthwashes like those made by Biotene.

3. Loss or Alteration of Taste or Metallic Taste in Mouth (Dysgeusia)

Changes in taste can be merely irritating, but can sometimes decrease your desire to eat, thus affecting nutrition. There is not a lot you can do about this, but here are a few suggestions to cope:

- Avoid foods with sweeteners because they can increase metallic taste.
- Add strong herbs to your cooking, such as basil, dill, coriander, oregano, rosemary, and thyme.
- Use a tongue scraper: it is inexpensive and can really help.

4. Burning Mouth Syndrome or Burning Tongue (Neurotoxicity)

This condition can make you feel as though you have been scalded by a hot drink. It can be a function of dry mouth and mouth sores, but no one really knows what causes it. It is also sometimes linked with anxiety or depression and, at other times, with nutritional deficiencies.

Burning mouth seems to happen in women more than men, and it can appear spontaneously. As with dry mouth or sores, it can become dangerous if it inhibits your ability to eat well or practice good dental care.

Here are some natural remedies for burning mouth:

- Suck on ice chips
- Try low-sugar, no-alcohol, and nonacidic sorbets like banana, watermelon, and cucumber sorbet. However, you should avoid these if your teeth are sensitive to cold.

5. Cavities (Caries)

The decreased flow of saliva during cancer treatment can cause cavities and tooth decay. This is best treated by keeping your mouth extra clean and avoiding sugar. Fluoride rinses can help too.

6. Sensitive Teeth (Dentinal Hypersensitivity)

Both chemotherapy and radiation may increase sensitivity. The best thing is to carry on with your usual routine for keeping your mouth clean as much as possible. Also, follow our tips for mouth sores. A toothpaste made for sensitive teeth can help too (see our Appendix).

7. Nutritional Problems

Poor nutrition and weight loss may result from eating difficulties caused by mouth sores, dry mouth, and altered taste. Alert your oncology team immediately if you feel you can't eat, as this can interrupt your treatment and lead to malnourishment.

8. Bisphosphonate-Induced Osteonecrosis (ONJ)

ONJ, a *very* serious complication of radiation, is the irradiated bone's reduced ability to heal due to reduced blood flow to bones after high-dose radiation. In severe cases, the bone can begin to die and break down, and can have disastrous consequences if the patient has to have oral surgery after treatment—such as a biopsy, tooth extraction, and so forth. ONJ most frequently occurs in the lower jaw.

Although radiation therapy to the head and neck is the most common culprits, chemotherapy drugs pamidronate (Aredia) and zoledronate (Zometa) are also associated with it. These are some of the symptoms:

- Jaw and/or gum pain
- Numbness, swelling
- Infection
- Loose teeth
- Pus flow from jaw
- Eroded gum tissue with visible eroded bone

Because ONJ can sometimes go unnoticed during treatment, it's very important to be screened for the condition *before* treatment and to have regular dental checkups while in treatment to monitor bone health.

Unfortunately, the risk of ONJ does not diminish with time and may be a lifelong issue. Dental implants appear to pose a higher risk. The treatments for ONJ are significant and can include surgery, bone grafts, and titanium plates to retain jaw continuity and functioning. Check with your oncology team and dentist for more suggestions on how to avoid ONJ.

9. Infection

Chemotherapy depresses the immune system, leaving it vulnerable to bacterial and viral infections that need to be dealt with immediately. Identifying and treating oral health issues before beginning treatment, getting a clean bill of health, and maintaining impeccable oral hygiene during treatment are a must to avoid complications by secondary infections. Dr. Michael Sinkin puts it simply: "A dental infection during aggressive chemotherapy can be life threatening."

10. Bleeding Mouth and Gums

Bleeding and tooth loosening from gums is a much less frequently reported side effect of cancer treatment, but this can result in tooth loss or jaw stiffening and loss of mobility (trismus or tissue fibrosis). See your dentist immediately if you experience these symptoms.

RECORD KEEPING.
As with any long-term or ongoing medical issue, "the importance of keeping good medical records cannot be overstressed," according to Dr. Steven Bornfeld. You will like be going from facility to facility for treatments, as well as being treated by several teams of doctors. Keeping a comprehensive, organized, and easily accessibly paper trail is extremely important for continuity of treatment as well as keeping all parties informed of issues that can arise. Plus it can set you at ease to know you have everything at your fingertips when needed.

DENTAL HEALTH AFTER TREATMENT

While mouth sores will likely subside several weeks to a month or two after your treatment ends, certain conditions may persist.

Dry Mouth

Dry mouth may be permanent if you received radiation. In this case, your teeth may be more susceptible to decay. Be extra vigilant with your oral care and get regular checkups to reduce the chance of cavities. Your dentist may wish to put you on a prescription high-fluoride gel for tooth brushing.

Swollen, Tender Gums or Numbness

Patients being managed for chronic leukemia often get swollen, tender gums. If you see a change in the appearance of your gums, alert your dentist or oncologist.

Dental Work after Cancer Treatment

In general, you should wait *at least four months after treatment* is over to have tooth extractions. Your dentist should have you begin antibiotics before the extraction to minimize the risk of infection, and the surgery should be done with minimal trauma. And don't forget to resume normal dental care!

FREQUENTLY ASKED QUESTIONS ABOUT DENTAL HEALTH

What chemotherapy drugs are most likely to cause issues?
Dr. Gregg Schneider offers this list:

- Antitumor antibiotics: Doxorubicin (Adriamycin, Myocet, Doxil, Caelyx); anticancer agents that interrupt the action of cell division, slowing the growth of cancer
- Antimetabolites: Cytosine arabinoside (Cytarabine); Methotrexate (Trexall); Fluorouracil, 5FU (Adrucil, Carac, Efudex and Fluoroplex); Capecitabine (Xeloda); anticancer agents that restrict the growth of rapidly reproducing cancer cells
- Alkylating agents: Cisplatin (Platinol), Melphalan (Alkeran), cyclo-phosphamide (Endoxan, Cytoxan, Neosar, Procytox, Revimmune); slow the growth of cancer
- Plant alkaloids or topoisomerase inhibitors: Etoposide (Toposar, VePesid, Etopophos); anticancer agents that attack cells at various points of division, slowing the growth of cancer
- Bisphosphonates: Aredia, Zometa, Fosamax, Boniva, Actonel, Atelvia, Reclast; this category of drug has raised concerns within the dental field

Dr. Steven Bornfeld adds: "Patients receiving hematopoietic stem cell transplantation (HSCT), a controversial treatment most often used to treat blood and bone cancers, multiple myeloma, or leukemia, may be at risk for oral complications."

At what point in my treatment cycle can I expect issues?
Dr. Michael Sinkin: "The most common oral manifestations of chemotherapy and radiotherapy are as follows:

- Dry mouth and mucositis start about the second week of treatment.
- Oral ulceration and taste alteration start in the second week.
- Bleeding gums, hypersensitive teeth, and radiation caries (cavities) are usually delayed onset, as is ONJ."

I am hearing more and more about how the mouth is the "gateway to health." Can you explain more?
Dr. Alina Krivitsky: "We are now learning that oral issues are not separate or distinct from other physical concerns; mouth sores, dry mouth, inflammation of the gums, and tooth decay can all be indicators of wider physical issues such are heart disease, diabetes, stroke, and premature birth. Dental health is critical to overall health. The June 2008 issue of The Lancet Oncology contains a study indicating that men with periodontal disease may be more likely to develop cancer than men with healthy gums....These study findings are significant in that they suggest that cancer is potentially another systemic disease state associated with periodontal disease. This study should particularly encourage men [and women] to be mindful of their teeth and gums now that gum disease may play a role in the onset of cancer."

What's the best way to clean my mouth during treatment?
Dr. Alina Krivitsky: "Use a mild flavor toothpaste with fluoride and alcohol-free mouth rinses. Salt rinses (one teaspoon of salt and two cups of water) should be used frequently if toothpaste cannot be tolerated. Swabbing oral tissues with gauze dipped in a chlorhexidine rinse can be used to remove particles. Avoid using products containing alcohol, hydrogen peroxide, or high pH (acidic). If mucositis occurs, it is recommended to see your dentist as soon as possible."

How often should I see my dentist during my treatment?
Renita Sansom, RDH: "We recommend that the patient see us every 3 months, or in some cases, even every 6 weeks or 2 months. Changes or problems are much easier handled early on in a patient with a weakened immune system, rather than when they are advanced and more involved.

Also, systemic health is a big concern and, when the bacteria level in the mouth is less, the whole body is healthier and the immune system stronger."

Will chemo change the color of my teeth?
Dr. Alina Krivitsky: "There is no evidence that chemotherapy *alone* directly causes tooth yellowing or discoloration. Tooth discoloration is usually caused by various factors such as cavities, stains, or plaque/tartar buildup. Also, some mouth rinses such as Chlorhexidine (used to treat other oral infections) may cause teeth staining if used on a long-term basis, say more than two weeks.

"And notably, it's very common for many people undergoing cancer therapy to prioritize dental appointments less than other medical conditions due to depression, difficulty with manual dexterity, or preoccupation with other medical issues. The best way to prevent any tooth issues is to have very frequent oral hygiene and follow up on dental cleanings and checkups at least every three months."

Is it necessary to start fluoride treatments before cancer treatment?
Dr. Harvey Shiffman: "Fluoride delivery trays are a necessity for protecting teeth when radiation is in the head and neck area, as salivary glands can be affected and reduced saliva leads to increased caries, gum disease, and infections."

My grandmother had all her teeth extracted before her radiation treatment. Does this mean I should expect to as well?
Dr. Steven Bornfeld: "Years ago, it was considered routine to extract all remaining teeth in patients scheduled to undergo radiation therapy to the head and neck. This is not as true as it once was—both because radiation therapy has improved in its ability to limit radiation exposure outside the therapeutic field and because the importance and availability of regular dental care is better-known.

"Nevertheless, one still hears occasionally of 'radiation caries,' which is often impossible to control, necessitating extractions. In patients who have had radiation to their jawbone, this is something to be avoided—even if it means sacrificing a few extra teeth beforehand."

Will cancer treatment ruin previous expensive dental work (porcelain veneers, crowns, etc.)?

Dr. Alina Krivitsky: "Not usually, but cancer treatment can have a detrimental effect on reduction of salivary flow (radiation therapy may cause temporary or permanent damage to the salivary glands, and some medications may cause salivary flow reduction), which may increase likelihood of [cavities]. As saliva is the first line of immune defense against intraoral bacteria, this may result in recurrent caries under *existing* dental restorations (crowns, fillings, veneers, etc.) or can predispose patients to root caries, which is a very fast deterioration process. What helps to prevent such effect is very diligent and more frequent oral hygiene at home as well as routine dental checkups and dental cleanings every three months—or even more often. Preventive use of fluoride rinses or gels may help slow down the caries process by helping with teeth remineralization."

Dr. Harvey Shiffman adds: "Chemo and radiation in and of itself does not damage dental restorations. Mucosal tissues become inflamed by chemo and radiation if the oral cavity or salivary glands are in the field can be affected. [Mouth sores] are common after and during chemo. This causes discomfort, and many patients do not adequately perform routine daily brushing and flossing, and they can develop dental caries and periodontal issues. Lidocaine rinses combined with Maalox-type preparations soothe the inflammations and help with comfort with hygiene and nutrition."

My doctor is talking about bisphosphonate therapy. What is this and will it affect my mouth?

Dr. Alina Krivitsky: "Intravenous bisphosphonate therapy is prescribed for patients with cancer that has spread to the bone to help decrease associated pain and fractures and possibly inhibit the spread of cancer to the bones.

Oral bisphosphonates taken for more than five years and bisphosphonates that are administered intravenously are particularly the subject of precautions for bisphosphonate-induced osteonecrosis [ONJ, or death of bone]... If a patient is receiving intravenous bisphosphonates or is taking oral bisphosphonates for over five years, invasive dental procedures should be avoided, unless absolutely necessary.

"Patients may be recommended to get a CTX (serum C-terminal telopeptide) test done. It is a medical blood test measuring bone turnover rate and is used to assess the risk of oral bisphosphonate-induced osteonecrosis of the jaws and guide treatment decisions... If patient falls into a high-risk category, [his or her] physician must be contacted to discuss possible 'drug holiday' (a physician-determined time period, where patient is taken off the bisphosphonates)." Your oncology team will be aware of this and guide you accordingly.

Can I get radiation-induced mouth issues even if I am protected by a lead apron?
Dr. Michael Sinkin: "Radiation therapy induces cell death and vascular changes to the exposed areas, which unfortunately is not limited to diseased tissue. Despite precautions, including the use of protective shields, healthy tissue will be irradiated and affected. Generally when it comes to head and neck irradiation, doses of 200cGy per week or greater have the most significant oral side effects, and long-term effects are most often seen when total dosage exceeds 3000cGy."

I'm terrified of developing mouth cancer now that I am going through treatment for another cancer. Any suggestions?
Dr. Harvey Shiffman: "We employ a device called the Velscope Vx oral cancer screening device as an aid to visual and tactile examinations. The Velscope works by visualizing the fluorescence differences between healthy and cancerous tissue...when the blue wavelength of light is exposed to the tissue, the difference is seen in the scope (looks kind of like night vision): healthy tissue appears pinkish green, while unhealthy tissue has a dark green to black appearance. The Velscope is an aid to diagnosis, which must be confirmed with a biopsy. Statistics show that the average dentist will diagnose

five cases of cancer in twenty-five years of practice. In the last two years using the Velscope, we have diagnosed five cases alone, one resulting in a loss of life. Previously we would screen patients fifty years and older, but now with the high incidence of head and neck cancers caused by the HPV virus, we have lowered the age to thirty and lower if the patient is overly sexually active." Ask your dentist if this screening might be for you.

My doctors mentioned "growth factors" that can help with mouth sores. Can you explain?
Dr. Steven Bornfeld: "Promising new biological therapies such as growth factors may speed recovery from painful mouth sores. These agents work in the opposite way to chemotherapy: instead of attacking and killing cells, they encourage the growth of healthy cells that line the mouth and GI tract. These include granulocyte colony-stimulating factor (G-CSF), granulocyte macrophage colony-stimulating factor (GM-CSF), epidermal growth factor, human keratinocyte growth factor (palifermin, brand name Kepivance), and transforming growth factor. Speak with your oncology team."

My friends who went through treatment tell me I'm definitely going to get horrible mouth sores. Isn't there anything I can take to prevent them?
Not usually. But according to the Oral Cancer Foundation if you're undergoing radiation, "midline radiation blocks and 3-D radiation treatment" may lower the risk of mucositis. For patients with head and neck cancer, benzydamine (a nonsteroidal anti-inflammatory also known as Tantum Verde) can help. If you're undergoing chemotherapy, the use of "ranitidine [Zantac] or omeprazole [Prilosec] to prevent epigastric pain after cyclophosphamide, methotrexate, and 5-fluorouracil or treatment with 5-fluorouracil with or without folinic acid chemotherapy" can help. Your oncology team should be aware of these options and guide you accordingly.

I like mints to moisten my mouth, but which are safe to eat?
Dr. Julie Goldstein: "Sugar-free mints may be effective in increasing salivary flow and providing relief. I prefer mints containing xylitol, which is not

cariogenic. Never use candy or mints containing sugar because the combination of decreased saliva and increased sugar can readily lead to tooth decay."

Can I still use my dental pick and toothpicks?
Dr. Mindy Hochgesang: "Discontinue use of toothpicks, which may introduce infection."

Any natural ice pop recommendations for my sore mouth?
Dr. Magali Chohan: "You can make homemade rose petal ice pops. A recent scientific study published in *Gastroenterology and Hepatology from Bed to Bench* shows that essential rose oil is able to kill human colon cancer cells in vitro. It's easy to harness the antioxidant and anti-inflammatory power in this easy-to-make and soothing treat. Because the effects of rose on chemotherapy are not known, ask your oncology team first and have these as an occasional treat.
You'll need:

- Culinary-grade rose petals
- Honey (optional)
- Ice pop molds and sticks

Place 1 gram of rose petals in a large mug with about 6 ounces of water, and place in a pan of water on the stove. (If you'd like to use honey, add about 1 tablespoon now.) Bring the water to a boil. Remove the mug from the heat and let infuse for five minutes. Strain the rose petals and allow the solution to cool. Add another cup of water to the mug and stir. Pour the liquid into the ice pop molds and allow to freeze for at least four hours. The popsicles will keep for a week.

What can help dry mouth?
Dr. Mindy Hochgesang: "I recommend Biotene as a saliva substitute. Drinking water and sucking on ice chips also relieves dry mouth. Additionally, I recommend chewing sugar-free gum with xylitol. This gum stimulates salivary

glands, and xylitol prevents cavities. The patient's dentist may suggest prescription toothpaste with higher fluoride content to prevent cavities."

I don't want to take a prescription mouth rinse. Any suggestions for a natural one?
Dr. Julie Goldstein: "You may find relief by rinsing with a solution of a half teaspoon salt and two tablespoons baking soda dissolved in four cups of water."

Is there anything I can use to ease pain before eating?
Dr. Steven Bornfeld: "Topical analgesics help combat pain and dysphagia when used prior to meals. These include Difflam (benzydamine hydrochloride), 2 percent Lidocaine solution mouthwash, and aspirin/Mucaine mouthwash (aluminium hydroxide, magnesium hydroxide, and oxethazaine)."

Do any herbs help with mouth sores?
Dr. Magali Chohan: "Rosemary and thyme have antioxidant, anti-inflammatory, antibacterial, and antifungal properties; using rosemary and thyme as a mouth rinse to gargle can be very useful to keep infections at bay. Adding marshmallow leaves, which are very rich in mucilage, may have a protective effect for the sores. Anecdotal reports have been positive with the combination of rosemary, thyme, and marshmallow mouthwash; however, no scientific studies have yet been carried out on the efficacy of this recipe."

My dry mouth from radiation has never gone away. It's not as bad as it was, but what can I do?
Dr. Chad Denman: "Oncology patients will continue to have dry mouth after treatment is completed, so use of the artificial saliva should continue [or begin, if it has not already]. I recommend patients suck on sugar-free candies like lemon drops to help restore their saliva flow naturally."

Can I floss?
Renita Sanson, dental hygienist, Dental Oncology Professionals (Garland, TX): "It is usually OK for a cancer patient to floss, but just as

a patient who needs to undergo oral surgery, we consider their history of present illness, their blood count, consultation with their oncologist, etc. As a general rule, in a patient whose immune system is not too compromised, gently flossing with waxed or tape floss is OK...again, as long as it is during times when they are not myelosuppressed. We recommend they participate in the fullest oral hygiene protocol tolerable and use an extra soft brush."

Is there anything to help regain my normal taste?
Dr. Alina Krivitsky: "The use of 220mg zinc sulfate supplements three times a day may help with recovery of taste."

Will I be able to wear my dentures after treatment is over?
Dr. Michael Sinkin: "Patients suffering from mucositis [mouth sores] as well as patients undergoing head and neck radiation often cannot wear partial or full dentures for a long period of time... If a patient's mouth has been irradiated, often dentures cannot be worn for months after therapy to avoid trauma to the underlying bone. For patients suffering from permanent xerostomia [dry mouth], denture use is problematic because moisture is an important factor in the prosthesis' fit. Denture adhesive is a big help as well as coating the mouth with K-Y Jelly prior to denture insertion."

What types of infection might I get?
Dr. Alina Krivitsky offer this list:
   "*Bacterial infection: Localized odontogenic* infection may be difficult to diagnose due to frequent lack of swelling; 25 to 54 percent of septicemia in cancer patients may originate from the oral cavity.
   Viral infection: Herpes simplex virus type I reactivation may occur. Prophylactic Acyclovir helps to effectively control viral infections. Other viruses such as varicella zoster virus (VZV), cytomegalovirus (CMV), Epstein-Barr virus (EBV), herpes viruses 2, 6, 7, and 8, and respiratory viruses can cause infections but are less common.

Fungal infection: Candidiasis is the most commonly occurring secondary infection in patients undergoing chemotherapy. It can cause burning sensation and taste alterations and interfere with swallowing. It can spread to esophagus systemically and can even cause infectious death. It can be treated with topical and systemic antifungal medications.

Thrombocytopenia: Decreased platelet number is a common complication. It puts patients at risk of postoperative bleeding after dental surgery when the platelet count is <50,0000/mm^3. Spontaneous bleeding can occur with <20,000/mm^3."

...so what might my dentist prescribe for an infection?
Dr. Alina Krivitsky: "For fungal infections systemic and topical antifungal medications (that is, fluconazole, amphotericin B, nystatin) are helpful. Bacterial infections can be treated with antibiotics (that is, bacitracin, vancomycin) and viral infections with antiviral medication (that is, Acyclovir, valacyclovir)."

DENTAL TIPS FROM SURVIVORS

"Take care of your teeth! I had three crowns put on after chemo. It is hard on teeth. During chemo, I found I could not tolerate regular toothpaste. A fellow cancer buddy gave me some Biotene toothpaste. It worked! No more gagging. Also after my first treatment of chemo, I had mouth and throat sores. I found out that drinking a cold drink or eating ice during chemo treatment saved me from this side effect for future rounds." —Lynn Jones

"I was diagnosed with stage 3 Diffuse B Cell non-Hodgkin's lymphoma... My treatments went fairly well [but] I had cankers along the inside of my cheeks, the insides of my lips, and on the sides of my tongue, which were painful...[lidocaine] mouth rinse helped, and I used it for quite a while after the chemo was over." —Martina Lavoie, www.breadsaltwine.com

"Use an oral irrigator to help crevices stay clean." —Eva Grayzel, author of the *Mr. C Plays Hide and Seek*

"I was given a prescription for Magic Mouthwash. Instead of swishing with it, however, I soaked a Q-tip in the solution and then dabbed it on specific sores. I also suggest following all advice about avoiding spicy food, salt, and citric acid, at least until after finishing the die-off phase." —Heidi Bright, M. Div. www.heidibright.com

CHAPTER SIX

MAKEUP AND STYLE

WITH ALL THE CHANGES, ISSUES, AND concerns that come with cancer diagnosis, makeup would seem to be the last thing you would care about. Yet cancer treatments bring on a whole slew of new challenges that can impact your face. Radiation and chemotherapy may cause changes in skin tone, dryness, dark circles under your eyes, or loss of eyebrows or eyelashes. Your face and lips may become thinner or fuller. You may have unexpected dark patches. In all these cases, makeup can become your best friend.

Maybe you have been wearing makeup since you were fifteen years old and know every trick in the book. Maybe you long ago decided that makeup was not your thing. Whatever the case for you, be open-minded. You do not have to spend hours viewing instructional videos or have to learn time-consuming techniques. With the right cosmetics, which do not have to be expensive, you can cover imperfections and brighten up your face. And since chemo and radiation can make you feel very tired, we introduce the "five-minute face" so you can get on with your day quickly and easily. Although playing with makeup can be fun, we will concentrate only on how to use makeup to address issues associated with cancer treatments.

As supermodel Cindy Crawford once said, "Even *I* do not wake up looking like Cindy Crawford." We all can use a bit of help, and this chapter shows you how.

MAKEUP

Stress, surgery, chemotherapy, and radiation can all impact your face and make you feel and look more tired than you are. Your skin texture and health may change (see below). Your skin tone may change too. You may look paler and ashy. Conversely, you can look tanned and red. You may also find you have dark spots or blemishes you wish to hide. Chemotherapy can cause weight *gain* as well as weight *loss*, and easy contouring to reduce or increase fullness can work wonders to make you look like you.

Makeup artist Fawn Monique identifies the most common issues you may experience:

- Changes in skin type: skin can become overly dry or oily or look aged, ashy, pale, or thinned
- Changes in skin tone: lightening, yellowing, darkening, hyperpigmentation, bruising, ashiness, reddening, or taking on a greenish tint
- Skin dulling: loss of radiance, a flat look
- Brow and eyelash release: can get sparse or total loss
- Dark circles and sunken eyes: any darkness is more pronounced and eyes can appear hollowed
- Whites of the eyes: some chemotherapy drugs can give your eye whites a bluish or yellowish tint
- Lips texture: can become very chapped
- Lip tone: lips can lighten or darken
- Face shape: can become fuller or thinner

Don't forget that feeling good is more important than how you look. Fawn reminds us: "There are visual changes during cancer treatment, but the one I focus on the most is the *feelings* of my client. It is very important for her to see herself still as beautiful as she has always been, if not even more beautiful as she goes through these treatments. It's important to keep your spirits up." This chapter shows some innovative makeup techniques from experts who have lots of experience working with women during treatment.

We have kept the information in this chapter short and sweet and stuck to just a few products and techniques for the most part; you may not feel like experimenting with tons of different products during healing.

EYEBROWS

"How your eyebrows look can make a huge difference in your appearance," states eyebrow expert Ramy Gafni. "Overly bushy brows can age you. Not having eyebrows at all can signal the world that you're going through chemotherapy." Whether your eyebrows have just thinned or released altogether, you can help achieve a beautiful look that minimizes your eyebrow changes with some makeup wizardry.

Pencil/Shadow

The easiest way to "fake" a brow is with makeup. Many makeup artists agree that powder eye *shadow* (not eyebrow powder) is the best way to go. Makeup artist Cindy Barbakov explains: "There is a much wider variety of eye shadow colors than there are eyebrow powders, so finding a good match is much easier." Used with an angled brush or a stencil, powder shadow can give a soft definition. But how do you get the most natural look?

- Learn from a pro: if you have no brows, makeup artist Dee Dee Jones-McCuen of Posh Pout suggests you see an expert first for a lesson: "It's worth the appointment to learn how to properly draw on an eyebrow and the appropriate thickness and color for the client's face."
- Practice: if you can't or don't want to see an eyebrow artist, Fawn suggests you practice your brows *before* you begin chemotherapy: "Practice shaping your existing brows by using an eye shadow powder and an angled brush. The brush is very important, as it does 80 percent of the work for you." Using your existing brow helps give you a sense of your face, so take a photo of yourself for future reference.
- Stencils: many makeup artists swear by stencils, and they come in a huge variety of shapes and sizes to suit your face shape. They can work beautifully, but they do require some practice to achieve symmetry.

- If you're wearing a wig, you may need to darken the eyebrow color a little to match the wig.

Brow Care during and after Chemotherapy—Tips from Brow Expert Ramy Gafni

- If your brows are thinning or releasing during chemo, do not remove a single hair. Once you finish treatment, don't keep trying to shape them into something. Be patient, and give your eyebrows a chance to grow back.
- Once your brows do start growing back, having them professionally shaped can make your brows look more substantial as they continue to grow in. Do not have them waxed or threaded. Go to someone who offers the more precise method of tweezing, and let them know you are recovering from cancer treatment.

Semipermanent Brow Treatments

Like the hair on your head, eyebrows will begin to regrow about two to three months after chemotherapy ends. But what can you do if they do not grow back in or grow in sparsely? Both semipermanent and more permanent solutions are available to you.

Henna tattooing: The same natural henna that can create the beautiful head crowns can also be used to mimic eyebrows. When used with a stencil, it can achieve a surprisingly natural look that will last five to seven days. Henna has the added bonus of not rubbing off, as some powders can. Henna kits are available on the Internet.

Semipermanent eyebrow tattooing: Permanent makeup—tattooing with semipermanent ink—has come a long way from the years of harsh black eye liner and penciled-on brows. New inks and techniques now create natural-looking brows that require very little maintenance. Julie Michaud, an expert in micropigmentation, uses a "hair-stroke" method to simulate real brows and achieve the most natural look. Be sure to find an expert in your area with amazing before and after photos: your local tattoo shop is not the place to go!

And consider timing: Julie says, "It's a good idea to have the procedure done *before* the hair loss begins so that the artist can follow the natural brow line. But even if not, always bring in photos so the artist can see what your brows looked like before the hair loss."

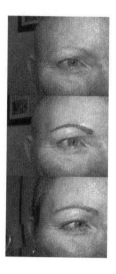

Eyebrow Tattoo, by Dr. Laura Reed

Latisse: Latisse can be a lifesaver and can be used on both lashes and brows combined. See below for information on its use for growing eyelashes. Latisse is available by prescription only, so see your dermatologist if interested.

Rogaine: Rogaine can be very helpful in regrowing brows. You just have to be careful not to apply it anywhere you don't want hair! See your dermatologist for more information.

Permanent Eyebrow Solutions

Eyebrow Transplantation: Like other hair transplant procedures, eyebrow transplantation uses follicles from the scalp which are then moved to the eyebrow area. After a few months, new eyebrows will grow in and the final, sometimes dramatic, result will be seen in 8-12 months.

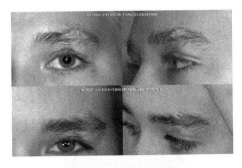

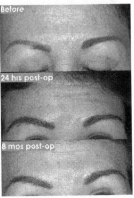

Eyebrow Transplantation by Dr. Alan J. Bauman

EYELASHES

Solutions using Makeup

If your eyebrows have become sparse or lost during treatment, it's likely your eyelashes have too. Fortunately, a defined lash line is easier to recreate than an eyebrow. If you've got some lashes, you can simply use mascara to define them. Try a thickening formula. Or sometimes you want to add a little more definition and drama to your eyes using false eyelashes. The trick is to use them carefully and sparingly (say, special occasions only). Here are more makeup tips from experts:

Fawn Monique: "Use a creamy eye liner that doesn't tug on your skin and a smudge brush to define your top and bottom lash line. Smudge the eyeliner to a level of color that you desire, and then set it in place with a powder eye shadow in the same color. A trick to remember for any makeup that wants to 'budge' is that powders always set creams."

Dee-Dee Jones-McCuen: "A nice little trade secret is to use a kohl pencil under the lash line, like the new one from Trish McEvoy. Flip up the lash line and draw in between the lashes to draw the eye upward and awake. This is a quick solution for someone with no lashes and a great volumizer for someone with little lashes."

Tim Quinn: "Boost the appearance of the lash line with a waterproof pencil on the lash line. You might try a deep brown...or be bold and wear color. Add a smudged line of shadow to soften the line. This looks more modern and helps draw attention away from the lash line."

Semipermanent Solutions

Eyelash extensions: If you want a more permanent solution to eyelash loss, you might try eyelash extensions. This sophisticated technique, which works like hair extensions to create volume and length, is rapidly growing in popularity. Courtney Akai was a pioneer in this field. She explains how extensions work and how they can help.

"Eyelash extension technique involves applying single synthetic or mink lashes at the base of your natural lash. There are lots of different lengths, from 6mm really natural-looking lashes to 15mm for full drama. The lashes come in various thicknesses and curl, making the result extremely personalized. Once selected, we apply the lashes one at a time using a specially formulated, semipermanent glue that will not irritate the eye or damage the natural lash. Applying a full-set of lashes takes about two hours and can be maintained year-round with touch-ups every three to four weeks. A half set of lashes can also achieve a dramatic effect economically.

"I can work with even the littlest of lash. Normally people have between 90 and 150 lashes. If a client is in chemotherapy, she may be down to twenty lashes. I can make that twenty look like about forty. A full set of extensions can also thicken them by 30 to 50 percent. What I do is crisscross the lashes to give a fuller look. I use a very lightweight lash in general and always a finer lash for cancer patients.

"Cancer patients should use fine silk or mink. Don't be put off by 'mink.' Nothing is done to the animal except shaving the hairs from the top of its coat. It's just like giving it a haircut, so it's humane, and the lashes are highly sanitized. If you're really against mink, you can always use a very thin synthetic lash. The key is to use as fine a lash as possible.

"These fine extensions don't add significant weight to the lashes and pull them down or cause them to fall out. Also, unlike traditional false eyelashes, the bonding agent does not touch the lash line or eyelid and therefore does not inhibit growth. We use three different types of pharmaceutical-grade bonding agents: all are made in United States and are ophthalmologist-tested. The glue is void of any toxic and/or cancer-inducing chemicals, including formaldehyde, a commonly used substance in adhesives.

"From start to finish, lashes will last about six to eight weeks. Because we understand the time and money factor, we apply each lash to the base of the natural lash, helping to maximize the length of time between touch-ups. We remove extensions with an organic solvent. It's very important that this is done by a professional so you don't inadvertently lose precious lashes by doing it yourself."

Latisse: As mentioned above, Latisse is a new topical cosmeceutical that helps grow eyelashes. Plastic surgeon Dr. Melissa Doft explains: "Latisse is a prostaglandin analog, indicated to treat hypotrichosis of the eyelashes by increasing their growth with regard to length, thickness, and darkness. I have had some patients who actually have to trim their eyelashes. Patients put it on at night to the skin directly under the upper eyelid margin. It is very easy." Over-the-counter alternatives to this prescription formula include Revitalash Advanced Eyelash Conditioner and neuLASH by Skin Research Laboratories Lash Enhancing Serum, says Courtney Akai.

Permanent Solution

Eyelash Transplants: If your eyelashes are not growing back after chemotherapy, you might consider eyelash transplants. This quick procedure uses your own transplanted hair follicles to create new lashes and permanently redistributes them into the eyelid. It is performed under local anesthetic and is purported to have just minor swelling. Sometimes eyelashes grow so long they need to be trimmed!

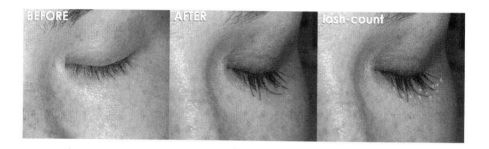

Eyelash Transplant Before and 12 Months After, by Dr. Alan J. Bauman

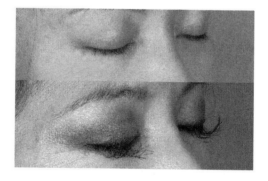

Eyelash Transplant, by Dr. Alan J. Bauman

DARK CIRCLES AND SUNKEN EYES

Purplish dark circles and eyes that appear more deeply set than usual are a telltale sign of any illness. Add to this weight loss, and you may develop a hollow look. Most makeup artists recommend you play up other parts of your face to distract attention from your eyes, but here are some tips and products to brighten the eyes up themselves:

Tim Quinn: "Try an eye cream, especially with light-reflecting quality. I love Giorgio Armani Beauty Crema Nera Reviving Eye Compact for this especially. Use a color corrector in the inner corners, like a rosy pink tone.

Blend with Giorgio Armani Beauty Maestro Eraser Concealer, which has a moonlight effect and also acts as treatment to help combat darkness. I like to apply on the lid as well to neutralize and discoloration. If you need more coverage, Clé de Peau makes a terrific, denser under eye concealer, as does Laura Mercier. I prefer using a synthetic concealer brush."

Fawn Monique: "If you have wrinkles under your eyes, some concealers can enhance that. You can break down your concealer by mixing it with a moisturizer or tinted moisturizer to get a thinner texture. This thins it but does not take away from the full coverage of the concealer. Using a layering effect can build to your desired level of coverage: pat on your concealer/moisturizer mix with a brush or finger, let it set for a moment, then go back in and place more product until you get the coverage you want."

Dee Dee Jones-McCuen: "A great under eye treatment/concealer is Instant Eyelift by Trish McEvoy. It makes even the darkest eyes lift up and beam! For extra coverage and brightening, add a highlighter like Touche Éclat by Yves Saint Laurent over it."

MAKEUP SAFETY

Krista Embry is a renowned makeup artist and the creator of Live Love Life, a program that helps women find themselves again during cancer treatment through hair and makeup techniques. Krista emphasizes safety. When your immune system is suppressed, you need to take every step to make sure you are not introducing extra bacteria into your system via cosmetics use. She recommends you put away your old makeup during treatment and buy replacements. Here are more of her tips:

- *Never, ever share makeup!*
- *To keep pressed eye shadows, powders, or other color palettes clean, use 70/30 alcohol to spritz palette. It will be clean and ready next time.*
- *If you use false eyelashes, use them occasionally and once only!*
- *Sharpen all pencils (eye and lip) after each use.*
- *Make sure you clean your brushes frequently. Synthetic brushes may be better for short-term use: they are less expensive and can handle more frequent washing.*
- *Try to use disposable mascara wands every time you apply.*
- *Cosmetic wedges are a must to keep foundations and other liquids from contamination. Use them once, then discard.*
- *Refrain from lining the inside of your eyes during treatment.*
- *Patch test any new products.*

CHANGES IN SKIN TONE

Chemotherapy can literally change your skin tone. Warm shades can become pallid; usually even tones can become overly rosy; and dark skin can take on ashiness. The good news is that once the chemicals clear your bloodstream, your complexion will begin to return to normal. In the meantime, think about *protecting*, *correcting*, and *perfecting* your skin.

Protect: Always moisturize and use a high-SPH sunscreen. Skin may be dry, and makeup does not work well on dry skin. If your skin is suddenly oily, broken out or irritated, see your dermatologist for help in determining the cause and treat with the appropriate formula.

Correct: If your skin tone takes on a greenish or bluish cast (like a bruise in areas), Fawn Monique suggests you use "color correctors such as yellow/green/violet, which help cancel out the hue. Then you can go on top with full coverage foundation to match to your skin tone."

Perfect: Most makeup artists swear by tinted moisturizer, which is light and undetectable. But sometimes foundation is more in order. Here are Fawn Monique's tips for giving your skin the texture and look *you* want.

For a dewy look, get sheer to medium foundation coverage with a tinted moisturizer and concealer (where needed). Dewy foundation adds a sheen to skin. You can balance that sheen by using a translucent setting powder to keep your face from looking overly moist throughout the day.

For a semimatte look, create medium coverage by using a sheer/medium foundation and concealer where needed. Set it with a mineral powder or translucent powder to keep your look all day.

For a matte effect, achieve medium to full coverage by using concealer where needed and then heavier foundation set with a powder to finish. Blending is very important with this more made-up look! If you get the look of too much powder or a cake-like residue, use a spray toner or water to counteract it: spray on your hands and gently pat into the skin to reduce the texture.

LOSS OF RADIANCE

Chemotherapy can literally suck the life out of your skin. Besides killing off cancerous cells, it dehydrates the body and diminishes the look of healthy skin. Drink more water, and fake a glow while you and your skin heals with these tips:

Tim Quinn: "Use a luminous foundation, that is, LSF [Giorgio Armani Luminous Silk Foundation], with a touch of luminizer blended in (our Fluid Sheers are terrific for this: #2 has a subtle champagne undertone that is quite flattering, also #10 to add a slightly golden warmer touch). Foundation primer helps as well, as it tends to act as a barrier so that the skin doesn't absorb the moisture from the foundation. A gel primer is great. I found self-tanners quite helpful during my chemo treatments. The L'Oréal Sublime Bronze line is fab, gradually adding color so not to look Oompa Loompa."

Dee Dee Jones-McCuen: "Get a fabulous spray tan at your local salon! That's my favorite trick of all. Versa Spa is fantastic. It is a self-service treatment in a private room available all over the country. Walk out looking like a bronzed goddess!"

Fawn Monique: "To add a bronzed look to your skin, bump up your normal foundation to a little deeper shade and use it in a thinner application, blending down to your neckline and décolleté. Sheer tinted moisturizers are great to do this with too, so you can easily add radiance and glow to the skin. Using a cream blush will add a pop of color to your cheeks."

CHANGE OF FACE SHAPE

When surgery or chemotherapy wreaks havoc on your weight, your face will show it. Chemotherapy weight gain can show in your face and eyes, and hormone therapy can cause water retention and puffiness. Conversely, you may lose weight and feel you look gaunt.

Highlighting and contouring can make a world of difference in the way you see your skin and face shape. You can take attention away from areas you might not be comfortable with and highlight those you like. This technique really depends on your face shape and what elements of your face you want to bring out or recede. Looking at visuals of different face shapes can determine your personal face shape and where you would place your light and dark tones.

If You Have Lost Weight...

If you've lost weight during your treatment, consider adapting how you put on your blush: put blush *only* on the apples of the cheeks, not under the cheekbones. This will give you a fresher look and a fuller, rounder appearance. Tim Quinn likes a cream blush because it can look more luminous. Krista Embry agrees: "It looks more natural and floats on skin rather than drying and looking cakey." You can use a tinted moisturizer with soft shimmer to add fullness too.

If You Have Gained Weight...

Krista Embry: "Use spray bronzer *without* shimmer: "Spray an A or a Z shape over your whole face and blend well."

Tim Quinn: "Sweep a bronzer across the temples at the cheekbone and along the jawline to add depth and dimension—think about making the shape of a three [3]."

If You Have Puffy Eyes...

Cindy Barbakov: "If you have time in the mornings, gently massage your eye area with ice cubes. Do it for about five minutes. It will make you look more awake, make the whites of your eyes brighter, and make under your eyes less puffy."

CHAPPED LIPS AND CHANGED LIP COLOR

Chemotherapy can cause your lips to be cracked, and you should moisturize throughout the day with an emollient balm or lip serum that contains an SPF. Dermatologist Dr. Cynthia Bailey cautions: "Avoid the seductive 'healing lip balm' ingredients that often get you addicted to lip balm; these ingredients can actually chap your lips, leaving your running for more lip balm. Use lip balms made from only the active moisturizing ingredients [like] shea butter." Other favorites are Aquaphor and La Mer lip balm.

Or you can try a homemade moisturizer like Dee Dee Jones-McCuen does: "Turn coconut oil into a skin treatment by mixing a few drops of essential oils with coconut oil and blend for several minutes in a food processor. This makes a rich body balm: it really is divine and feels like an expensive luxury cream!"

Dry lips can affect lipstick application, leaving clinging bits of skin or obvious lines; give your lips moisture so your lipstick will wear better. If your lips are very dry, avoid shiny lip gloss, which can highlight the dryness, as well as traditional matte finish lipsticks, which can make it worse. Try exfoliating your lips with a natural sugar scrub, and then apply lip balm. Let the lip balm sit for a few minutes before applying lipstick.

To apply lipstick, you can use the traditional lip liner/lipstick technique, or you might like to soften lipstick by dabbing with your finger to create the shape. Cindy Barbakov says: "The color will look more natural, and the pressing action will grind its pigment onto your lips for staying power."

QUICK LOOKS

You may find the third and fourth day after a chemotherapy treatment to be extremely exhausting. Standing even ten minutes to apply makeup becomes a chore. We asked some pros to show us their quickest beauty routines for the days you have very little energy for much of anything, much less "doing your face."

Tim Quinn's Five-Minute Face

1. Moisturize. I like to add a few drops of Giorgio Armani Beauty Fluid Sheer Luminizer for a bit of glow.
2. Use an eyebrow pencil to frame your eyes.
3. Put waterproof brown eyeliner on your lash line—particularly if you have lashes.
4. Blend rose-toned cream blush onto the apples of your cheeks.
5. Use sheer lip moisturizer with a "pop" of color: I love Clark's Botanicals Lip Tints that come in tubes.

Ramy Gafni's Five-Minute Face

1. Perfect your complexion. Apply a concealer that matches your skin tone exactly around entire orb of your eyes—below the eyes and from lash line to brow bone. Then add the concealer where needed on face

to perfect your complexion: nasal folds, blemishes, red marks. Blend well using your fingertips or a sponge.

2. To choose your best shade of concealer, apply it along your jawline. Give it a minute to set. If you can't see the swatch of concealer, it's your perfect shade. If you can see the concealer, it's too light, too dark, or has the wrong undertone for your skin. Use where needed.

3. Set the concealer with translucent pressed powder.

4. Line upper lash line with brown/black eyeliner. Add black mascara to upper lash line only.

5. Add a neutral eye shadow to crease of eyes or onto eyelid.

6. Sweep powder blush onto apples of cheeks, blending upward.

7. Add lip color.

8. If you want to simplify this routine further, skip the eye shadow, blush, and lip color and opt for a multiple-use product instead to add color to your eyes, cheeks, and lips, such as Ramy Face Glosses.

FREQUENTLY ASKED QUESTIONS ABOUT MAKEUP

I choose to show my bald head, but am having trouble with matching my foundation with hair line now that it's exposed. What can I do?
Tinted moisturizer may be easy to work with and blends nicely into your hairline without being obvious. Makeup artist Andrea Charles suggests you can avoid the problem altogether: "A simple way to blend in foundation with your hair is to always apply foundation on your lower face using your finger, sponge or foundation brush, but avoid applying any foundation to the top half of your forehead and to the side of your temple and upper jaw where your hairline starts." Tip: make sure your foundation *exactly* matches your face.

My lips are cracking very badly, and I'm worried it's more than dryness.
Dr. Noëlle Sherber: "If cracking persists—particularly at the corners of the mouth—a dermatologist should check that there isn't a yeast infection,

called perleche. For perleche, a prescription anti-yeast anti-inflammatory ointment called Mycolog II works wonders—in a pinch, over-the-counter nystatin cream can be mixed into Aquaphor."

I usually wear bright lip color. But it looks like too much now that my lips are darker!
Fawn Monique: "Use a concealer or tinted moisturizer in either your skin tone or a shade lighter all over the lips to reduce their 'new' color, then apply lip liner/lipstick in the color desired. This is an easy way to get the true color of lipstick in the tube if your lips now have a lot of pigment. For example: your natural lip tone has a lot of bright red (like a cranberry), and you want to wear a coral lip color. You place it on, and it becomes a deep red orange vs. the coral tone you see in the tube. This is the time you would use the nuding effect on your lips to get the true of the color."

How do I get the best brow shape for my face?
Fawn Monique has some suggestions:

- Brows should begin diagonally up from the nostril, but consider how broad the nose is. For broader noses, go in slightly farther. Also consider the eye set. For close-set eyes, go out slightly farther.
- Your brow arches should be at the half or two-thirds point of the entire length. Brows should end diagonally from the end of nostril out.
- How high or low should the arch of your eyebrow be? Consider all your features and practice to avoid an angry or surprised look.
- How thick or thin should the brows be? If they are too thick, they may overpower the face; if they are too thin, they may look too severe. Look for a happy medium.

Makeup artists suggest a five-minute face routine, but sometimes I can't even manage that! Any suggestions?
Yes! Makeup artist Andrea Charles offers this two-minute, super-low-effort look:

1. Apply moisturizer of your choice
2. Pat on a light coat of powder.
3. Add powder blush.
4. Apply bright lipstick.
5. Finish with chic oversize sunglasses.

Can I safely use false eyelashes?
Dee Dee Jones-McCuen: "Gluing on lashes isn't dangerous. The trick is gently setting them atop the lash line onto the skin. It can be tricky and takes practice, but a lot of the waterproof glues stay on well. Of course, you must be more careful when wearing them: no rubbing eyes, etc. If you are allergic to latex, please take note: some eyelash glue contains latex and may irritate your eyelid skin, especially during treatment. Always read ingredients before using and choose the appropriate glue." For many makeup artists, the preferred brand of false eyelashes is Ardell.

Can I wear waterproof mascara during my treatment?
Yes, if you use a highly effective eye makeup remover to avoid excessive tugging at your lashes.

Hot flashes from hormone therapy are making my face shiny and my usual matte foundation is patchy!
Krista Embry: "The first thing to do is examine what you're putting on your face: be sure the products you use are free of petroleum and heavy oils. Skin can't breathe with heavy products, and perspiration will be trapped, making your skin worse. Try tinted moisturizer to even your skin out and follow with a light powder to set."

What can I do in a pinch if I don't have my lip balm with SPF?
Dr. Jeanine Downie: "Just use regular sunscreen for the face rubbed into lips and seal it in with a coat of Vaseline or Aquaphor."

Which are some makeup artists' favorite tinted moisturizers?
Dee Dee Jones-McCuen likes those by Laura Mercier; Ramy Gafni suggests a product from his own line, Sleep In Beauty.

I would like to add some color with a bronzer.
Tim Quinn recommends Hampton Sun Sunless Tanning Gel to give some color, or try Ramy Sun Smooched Bronzers.

My skin is so sallow. Can a primer help?
Ramy Gafni: "Primer is best used to create a smoother surface so that makeup goes on more evenly and lasts longer. That said, a primer like my Elixir Skin Conditioning Primer has a healthy dose of pure cucumber oil, which helps sooth irritation and redness. Then apply a tinted moisturizer or BB cream. They are sheer, so they are lightweight but they can counteract sallow coloring. You could try Ramy Sleep in Beauty tinted moisture cream, for example. Add a pale pink blush (mauve for olive skin, plum for dark skin tones) onto cheeks and over eyelids to further brighten while counteracting sallowness."

Tim Quinn: "A primer that has blue and pink pearlite like Giorgio Armani Beauty Master Primer helps blur imperfections as well as brighten sallow skin tones."

I would rather use a brow pencil than powder. Any tips?
Andrea Charles: "Always begin with a clean face. Make sure you have no lotion on your eyebrows. Use a brow pencil with a waxy consistency, which is more long-lasting. I sometimes use a little brow powder over pencil to help it to stay on longer and give a fullness, glow, and prettier look."

Can I still use my eyelash curler during treatment?
Not a good idea, says Dee Dee Jones-McCuen: "Stay far and clear of eyelash curlers during treatment. Lashes are sensitive and can be loosened and fall out."

MAKEUP TIPS FROM SURVIVORS

"No matter how poorly I felt, I made sure to put on organically based makeup and got out of my pj's each morning. It helped me so much mentally when I would look into the mirror each day to not see a 'sick' person" —Ivelisse Page, www.BelieveBig.org

"Taking care of ourselves during treatment is so important, and that means dressing like we always do, fixing ourselves up, and taking pride in our appearances. It did make a difference and all the compliments on how good a person looks—it's uplifting and continues to give you hope, and you need that when facing any cancer diagnosis." —Allison Sharpe

"Take the time to do your makeup if that was something that you did before. Cancer and its treatment will take so much out of you in and of itself. If you are feeling yucky and ill and then on top of that you're seeing yourself with no makeup, it will make you think that you look even worse." —Angelique Neumann, founder of RN Cancer Guides, www.rncancerguides.com

"During my treatment I came up with an inexpensive way to feel pampered. I went into the local department store and looked for a counter where the saleswomen seemed nice. I told them, 'Look, I can only afford to buy something small, but I have gone through a lot and would like to treat myself.' Contrary to what I expected, these ladies bent over backward. I went home with my purchase and a whole bag of samples to play with. Now I have some 'toys' in the medicine cabinet just for me and without any guilt. I learned: people want to help and you need to give them the opportunity to help. In doing so, you help yourself." —Mary A., five-year survivor

"As women, we all put ourselves behind the family, whatever our family might be. Some of us have kids, some don't—but we all usually have someone or something to care for when diagnosed. This is then the problem. The women who have just been diagnosed and finished in their first hospital stay, first lot of chemo or treatment, get home to a house longing for housework, kids wanting Mum to play and a husband/partner wanting to have some affection. The last thing on her mind is giving anything of herself—all she wants to do is sleep. Pampering or looking after herself is like number 500 on her to-do list and to her family, after all, she looks well. But do it! —Jodie Guerrero, activist and author of *Jodie's Journey*

"Latisse was prescribed for me to help retain my lashes during chemo. After I put the formula on my lashes, it was suggested I ran the brush across the brows, as it may help to retain them longer. It seemed to work, as I did not lose them until my last round of chemo and they grew back in less than two weeks." —Suzanne Flavin

"After treatment, my eyebrows really didn't come back strong, so I had them tattooed on, and it was like instant face-lift! My daughter lives in San Francisco and heard of a master technician in Chinatown and made an appointment. It was the best thing I ever did. I also used Latisse to grow long lashes, because again, my eyelashes didn't come in as thick." —Cindy Giles, cancer coach

"I put my makeup on as I always did…I blended well, and if I was not wearing a scarf on my bald head, no one would have known that I was going through chemotherapy. I looked like I always did. I did get pale when my blood counts lowered, so I wore less blush and blended—I did not want bright rosy cheeks with an all-paler face. I used the same colors—just less." —Allison Sharpe

"My number one tip—always wear makeup! It will make you look and feel better.

- Buy eyebrow stencils—it makes it so much easier.
- Use a makeup primer—your skin is dry and everything absorbs into it.
- Change to cream blush if you wear powder.
- Use eyeliner if you lose your lashes—it makes your eyes look normal." —Aileen Gold

"During and after chemo I found my brows and lashes were more sparse. I felt faded. Powdered eyebrow liner and angled brush were suggested. I still really like using powdered eyebrow liner, as it gives a softer, more natural brow and I can control the shape and how heavy I apply.

"As for lashes, a mascara with a small bristle wand gets all the small lashes, and an eyelash primer helps too. I like a hypoallergenic brand and often wear waterproof when going all day, especially when a sport is involved." —Mary Fedor, seven-year survivor

"I think the best eyebrow tattoos are those that have brush strokes woven into the tattoo. They look more natural. I am very fair skinned so I did not want to go very dark, even though they tell you the tattoos may fade over time. I'm pleased with color. Here are a few suggestions I'd make for someone getting them done though.

- Do your homework before choosing a tattoo artist. Look at some of their previous work and ask if you can speak to some of their clients. (Don't be shy—tattooing is permanent!)
- Take a friend with you on the day of getting it done. I didn't do this and really wish I had. I was nervous and when the artist showed me how it was going to look, I just wanted it over. Your friend will be your voice if yours is stifled. Mine are not exactly symmetrical (not bad, but not as good as they could be—they now have 'character').
- Make sure the tattoo artist has a fix-it or touch-up policy. As I type this, I am reminded that I can go back and have her even things up a bit at no charge." —Lynn Jones, author of *The Invisible Rocking Chair* (www.theinvisiblerockingchair.com)

"My Five Minute Face (Lana Koifman)

1. Apply tinted sun block to your face.
2. Tap on concealer or brightener under the eyes, such as Touche Éclat by Yves Saint Laurent.

3. Apply some blush. I liked Orgasm by Nars.
4. Dust the whole face with a mineral powder.
5. Apply very light eye shadow and a quick coat of mascara.
6. Finish with lipstick. She adds: "I often chose red—because you are fierce and everyone should know it!"

"The nurses told me that some of the chemo drugs could possibly cause a red mask on my face. Since I am fortunate to have a nice complexion before chemo, I had been able to use a moisturizer with a tint as my foundation, but I realized that to look as healthy as possible, I would need to use a more traditional foundation. So I went to a local makeup store, explained my situation, and they recommended a lightweight foundation in the right color. I did have a 'red' area from my cheeks over my nose each week I had chemo. The foundation covered it beautifully." —Suzanne Flavin

"If you have dry eyes, try Genteal eye gel. It's thicker than drops and distributes better in your eyes. Also, switch to glasses instead of contacts before starting chemo." —Dawn A. Gum

"Makeup tips:

- Use brown eyeliner to define your eyes and a lighter taupe eye shadow, applied with a small brush, to create eye brows.
- Keep your makeup to a bare minimum and use tons of moisturizer. A drop of liquid makeup mixed with moisturizer creates a healthy glow.
- Pink stick or gel blush on your cheeks, forehead, and chin can give you a sun-kissed glow no matter what skin tone you have.
- Then spray your face with an atomizer of water to set your makeup. Small cans of Evian spray can be bought in department stores, or you can make your own using purified water in a spray bottle.
- Your face is already dry, so you may choose to avoid face powder. It has a tendency to settle into cracks and, yes, crevices; the result of dehydrating treatments.

- My lipstick choice during treatment was Cover Girl Outlast Smoothwear. Once applied, you won't need a touch-up, even after eating. That little bit of color on your face can make such a difference.
- There is no makeup that can brighten your face like a smile. Beauty is only skin deep, but your smile comes from the soul. During treatment I even practiced smiling in the mirror for 'muscle memory' and used it when I felt like a wet noodle." —Kathleen O'Keefe-Kanavos, author of *Surviving Cancerland: The Intuitive Aspects of Healing*

"Before [your eyelashes thin], find a pair of false eyelashes that work for you and practice applying them. I also made a template of my eyebrows before I lost them so I could draw them in and have them look fairly normal. Here's how: take some tracing paper and trace the outline of each brow and mark how far away from your nose each one is. Then transfer that information to a clear plastic sheet and cut out the traced area of the brow. Make sure you transfer the nose markings too so you can position the template correctly on your face. Cut the sheet down to a size that fits over your brow area but is small enough not to cover your eyes. Then when you need to, you can position the template on your face and fill in your brow areas with a brow pencil—light feathery strokes and brush to blend." —Dawn A. Gum

"When I lost my eyelashes, I didn't wear mascara for a long time because I didn't want it to damage what few lashes were left. To 'fake' mascara, use a dark gel eyeliner." —Holly J. Bertone, author of *Coconut Head's Cancer Survival Guide* (www.coconutheadsurvivalguide.com)

"One thing that did work well for me when my eyelashes started to grow back was L'Oreal Telescoping mascara. The small applicator 'picked up' my fine lashes and made them seem longer and fuller. I still use it." —Sue Straatman

"One thing I wasn't prepared for was the loss of my eyebrows. The brows take a little longer to fall out than the rest of your hair, so start filling them in every day even though they are still there. That way, you become comfortable drawing the appropriate shape, and when they do start actually falling out you will already be used to drawing them." —Jessica Willey

"Get makeup tips from a drag queen. Seriously! They know how to contour, create illusion and magic. If you don't personally know one, watch *RuPaul's Drag Race* for inspiration. Embolden yourself with makeup: try a new lipstick you once thought was too bright or do a smoky eye just to run errands." —Jenny Saldaña, comedian

STYLE

During cancer treatment fashion may feel very unimportant, but you will feel much better if you are comfortable *and* look put together. Some days wearing loose sweatshirts or cuddly hoodies is entirely appropriate; however with a little planning, you can look great throughout your treatment with minimal fuss and discomfort, even on the days you are most exhausted. This brief section will give tips from style experts about choosing go-to outfits, giving yourself a lift with color, comfort and style during breast reconstruction, and must-haves for your wardrobe.

Style during Reconstruction and Other Surgery

Healing from surgery can take a while and present certain fashion challenges, particularly when it is a surgery that changes the shape of your body. Here are some suggestions from celebrity stylist Colin Megaro:

- Select items of clothing that float away from the body. A baby doll or empire waist can help disguise your chest area during the healing process.
- Buy clothing one size up and have a piece tailored inexpensively. By doing this you can create pieces to play up your assets and allow the extra room you need in sensitive areas.
- Avoid pants/skirts that are fitted or zippered if you experience swelling and weight change. Opt for pieces with stretch, a smooth waistband in the front, and elastic in the back.

- Choose clothing that doesn't wrinkle easily. During recovery you will be resting during the day, and it will be easier not to have to change outfits after.

Here are some more tips from stylist Jennifer Manghisi, a young breast cancer survivor:

- Don't be afraid of pieces with some stretch. These pieces can change with your body as it changes throughout reconstruction, and you don't have to buy clothing again and again.
- For many women, jersey fabric is a great choice: it is very comfortable, fitted but not too tight, and can be dressed up or down very easily. Many designers have jersey pieces that are convertible, meaning they can be worn in different ways. This feature is especially important if you are undergoing delayed reconstruction and have temporary breast asymmetry. Norma Kamali, Diane von Furstenberg, Donna Karan, and Calvin Klein all have jersey dresses in different styles and shapes.
- Another key piece during the reconstruction process is a sports bra with individual cups and full coverage but *no* underwire, which can irritate the skin. I like the sports bras with cups because you can stuff the cups with tissue in the event that your breasts are not quite the same size yet.
- Consider wearing a black top if you have had breast surgery. Black plays down the chest area, and you can have more confidence that you will not reveal too much about your surgery when tackling your day.

Fashion Go-Tos

The easiest way to make sure you can look good at any point in your treatment is to create a few "go-to" outfits. These can be as simple as an easy-fitting dress and loose blouse and slacks. The key is that the pieces are comfortable, stylish, easy to put on, light on the body, make you feel good. Take a few moments each night to make sure your outfit is ironed and ready to go.

Keep the colors neutral and the fit easy. This way you can throw on a scarf or other accessories and go. You will feel put together and more in control.

Post Treatment

After your treatment, you may wish to celebrate your new normal with some new pieces for your wardrobe, particularly if your body has changed due to surgery. Here is a checklist from celebrity stylist Colin Megaro to get started:

- A well-tailored white and/or black blouse.
- A well-tailored, chic suit. Buy a suit that has a jacket, skirt, *and* slacks. That way you get the best "bang for your buck." If you can't afford to purchase all three at the same time, pick a designer who uses similar fabrics each season. That way you can add to your wardrobe when you want.
- A great pair of jeans.
- Accessories. Continue to use the beautifully colored scarves you may have worn during cancer treatment. Easy-to-put on bracelets add the right pop to any outfit, and handbags with interior features like zippered pockets and slots for your phone can make your day easier.
- The perfect coat. Depending where you live, this may range from an overcoat to a trench. Remember to use it is as a layering/finishing piece and to pick one that works for your life. Easy-care, wrinkle-resistant fabrics go a long way in making it easy to be fashionable.

It's easy to find these pieces even with a small budget. There are great "spend-friendly" designers in every category and inexpensive tailoring always makes a piece look more finished and made for you.

Frequently Asked Questions

I had above-the-neck surgery and would love to hear some tips from a survivor to help with that area.
Childhood cancer survivor Marsha Danzig and author of *Fierce Joy*, used the "detract and accentuate" method, excerpted here from her book:

- Hermes silk scarf wrapped neatly around the neck, draping just so over my décolleté
- Tight black dress
- Massive Elsa Peretti [or other statement ring] glaring from right middle finger
- Chanel Red lipstick.

I just had breast reconstruction. How do I manage perspiration and irritation between my breasts under my bra while healing?
Try a bra liner such as Pambras, which are used at Memorial Sloan-Kettering Cancer Treatment Center. Liners like these are made of soft cotton to absorb perspiration and reduce rash-causing moisture and irritation from underwires and other bra features.

What do you recommend to even out my breasts during the expansion process?
Lana Koifman: "If you are going through a breast reconstruction, especially on one side, your breasts maybe different sizes during various stages of reconstruction. Silicone Breast Forms by Emson are terrific. They are light, and one size fits all. Put them inside the bra to correct the size of one breast."

Can you give some suggestions about inexpensive but nice clothing choices after my healing?
Celebrity stylist Colin Megaro:

Dresses
- Charter Club, three-quarter-sleeve cashmere sweater dress
- AGB dress, three-quarter-sleeve printed faux wrap
- Anthropologie convertible jersey dress

Tops
- a.n.a long-sleeve two-pocket shirt (JCPenney)
- Worthington long-sleeve satin-trim tunic top (JCPenney)
- St. John's Bay pintuck henley tee (JCPenney)

Pants
- Larry Levine crepe print pants with stripe
- Gap Pure Body pants
- Black House/White Market full-length legging

Pajamas
- Lauren Ralph Lauren pajamas, brushed twill notch collar top and pajama pants set
- Charter Club petite pajamas, brushed knit top and pajama pants set
- Miss Elaine long nightgown, brushed back satin

Handbags and Accessories
- Nixon Guide courier bag (available at Zappos)
- Juicy Couture Sophia Collection Essential Tote (available at Zappos)
- Croft & Barrow Essentials Shopper (Kohl's)
- Banana Republic turquoise pendant necklace
- Banana Republic gumdrop necklace
- White House/Black Market floral oblong scarf

STYLE TIPS FROM SURVIVORS

"Work out a treatment 'uniform' that you can wear. I was struggling with rapid weight gain and major financial issues, so I ended up living in sweats from the Goodwill. As I gradually began to get back on my feet, I read a lot about beauty and dressing the body you have now. I think the whole treatment experience would have been a little less difficult if I had chosen a few 'looks' that were very comfortable but flattering." —Rebecca Bogart, concert pianist and author of "From Chemo to Carnegie" at rebeccabogart.com

"Get out of your pj's and sweats and put on real clothes. Even if it's jeans and a shirt, being dressed like a normal member of society is a good trick to play on your mind and get you out of the 'I am sick' rut. When you take a few minutes every day to take care of yourself, you are going to feel better about yourself. I rocked those hats and scarves like no one's business. I was also a germaphobe during chemo and went everywhere wearing these cute little black gloves with bows on them so I didn't have to touch common surfaces with germs. Fortunately, it was winter, so it worked." —Holly J. Bertone, author of *Coconut Head's Cancer Survival Guide* (www.coconutheadsurvivalguide.com)

"Although I wore four-inch heels to every treatment, I suggest that you wear comfortable shoes. Do not wear shoes that pinch or cut into your foot. Open cuts can cause a serious infection." —Lana Koifman

"Wear something to chemotherapy that makes you feel empowered. I wore heels and a head wrap to my chemo treatments, and it's one of the best stories I can share. Also, bring a sweater because you may get cold during treatment." —Marlena Ortiz, young survivor and founder of Beating Cancer in Heels (www.beatingcancerinheels.org)

"The main area of discomfort I had was that during chemo, anything that pressed on my abdomen at all made me feel nauseous. Looking back, I could have done floaty empire tunics and leggings, or dresses and leggings." — Rebecca Bogart

"Don't be afraid to dress up. It doesn't matter if people can see your scars, if you're without breasts or even hair. Put on your favorite outfit and you'll get tons of reassuring compliments." —Angelique Neumann, founder of RN Cancer Guides, www.rncancerguides.com

"Super-padded nude bras create a great illusion even when you have nothing to insert. Also, anything worn on the neck such as necklaces or scarves will distract people from your chest area." —Marlena Ortiz

"Don't change your style during treatment! You are still you, no matter what cancer brings." —Lana Koifman

"If you're experiencing hot flashes, layers are the way to go during the day. The first layer to use is wicking. Then, a blazer or cardigan so you don't have to take off a layer over your head when you need to take off the top layer. Open-toe shoes year round. Sounds crazy in winter, but peep toe shoes are a hot-flashing woman's breath of cool air." —Haralee Weintraub, founder of Haralee.com, Cool Garments for Hot Women!

"Try to carry smaller purses with fewer things in them. If you are tired, you do not want to lug things around." —Lana Koifman, Surviving Beautifully founder

"Bring or wear something you *love* to your treatment: I rocked a feather boa. Buy something you've always wanted but always denied yourself (even if it's the cheap version)! For me, it was a pair of designer sunglasses. They're great hiding the 'bald' eyes and to keep the paparazzi away!" —Jenny Saldaña, comedian

CONTRIBUTING EXPERTS

Please visit our website, www.survivingbeautifully.com, for full biographies of many contributing experts.

DERMATOLOGISTS

Cynthia Bailey, MD. Dr. Bailey is a board-certified dermatologist in Northern California and the director and founder of Advanced Skin Care and Dermatology Physicians, Inc. She divides her professional focus between her full-time dermatology practice and writing about skin health for her acclaimed website and blog. To learn more about Dr. Bailey, visit www.drbaileyskincare.com.

Fredric S. Brandt, MD. Dr. Brandt is a board-certified internist, board-certified dermatologist, and one of the world's most renowned beauty experts. A pioneer in the use of injectables, he is the author of *10 Minutes 10 Years* and *Age-Less: The Definitive Guide to Botox, Lasers, Peels and Other Solutions for*

Flawless Skin. Dr. Brandt also dispenses his highly sought-after skin-care and beauty advice on his own Sirius XM Radio show, "Ask Dr. Brandt." To learn more about Dr. Brandt, visit www.drfredricbrandt.com.

Jeanine B. Downie, MD. Dr. Downie is a nationally recognized board-certified dermatologist practicing in New Jersey and the author of *Beautiful Skin of Color.* Dr. Downie has professional affiliations and lectures on behalf of some of the most prestigious medical societies, including the American Society for Dermatologic Surgery, the American Academy of Dermatology, the Women's Dermatologic Society, and the Skin Cancer Foundation, and she frequently appears in the media. To learn more about Dr. Downie, visit www.imagedermatology.com.

Debra Jaliman, MD. Dr. Jaliman is a world-renowned board-certified dermatologist with a private practice in Manhattan. For over twenty-five years, she has taught dermatology at Mount Sinai School of Medicine. She is the author of *Skin Rules: Trade Secrets from a Top New York Dermatologist* (2012). Dr. Jaliman was one of the first physicians to use Botox in her practice, and her office remains a national training center for Allergan, where she guides physicians on proper injection techniques. She frequently appears as an expert in the media. To learn more about Dr. Jaliman, visit www.drjaliman.com.

Tanya Kormeili, MD. Dr. Kormeili is a board-certified dermatologist in private practice in Santa Monica and clinical professor of dermatology at the UCLA School of Medicine and has authored numerous textbook chapters and articles on dermatology. A frequent speaker to both her industry and the public, Dr. Kormeili has been featured on television as well as in print and online media. To learn more about Dr. Kormeili, visit www.drkormeilidermatology.com.

Noëlle Sherber, MD. Dr. Sherber is a board-certified dermatologist in practice in Washington, DC, and a world-renowned expert in aesthetic and medical dermatology. Harvard-educated and Johns Hopkins–trained, Dr. Sherber has served as consultant dermatologist to the Johns Hopkins Scleroderma Center. She is considered a world authority in the skin manifestations and treatment of this disease. She is also prominently featured in the media. To learn more about Dr. Sherber, visit www.sherberandrad.com.

Anca Tchelebi-Moscatello, MD. Dr. Tchelebi-Moscatello is a medical aesthetician and board-certified radiation oncologist. She founded Park Avenue Medical Spa as a one-of-a-kind spa offering cutting-edge skin treatments, bioidentical hormone replacement therapy, and hair restoration. Dr. Tchelebi-Moscatello is a member of the American Academy of Medical Aesthetics and American Academy of Mesotherapy. To learn more about Dr. Tchelebi-Moscatello, visit www.parkavenuemedicalspa.com.

Shannon Trotter, MD. Dr. Trotter is a board-certified dermatologist with a special interest in skin cancer. She is assistant clinical professor and director of Pigmented Lesion Clinic at Ohio State University in addition to practicing privately. To learn more about Dr. Trotter, visit http://cancer.osu.edu/patientsandvisitors/findadoc/Pages/search.aspx?DocID=075192.

DENTISTS

Steven Bornfeld, DDS. Dr. Bornfeld has practiced in Brooklyn since 1977. He was formerly a clinical instructor in operative dentistry at NYU College of Dentistry. He is a member of the American Dental Association and the Academy of General Dentistry and a frequent contributor to various web dental and health forums. To learn more about Dr. Bornfeld, visit www.dentaltwins.com.

Chad Denman, DDS. Dr. Denman is a general dentist performing most specialist procedures, such as implants, root canals, wisdom teeth extractions, pediatrics, bone grafts, and sinus lifts. He is a member of the American Dental Association and Academy of General Dentistry. Dr. Denman practices in Austin, Texas. To learn more about Dr. Denman, visit www.familytreedentalgroup.com.

Julie K. Goldstein, DDS. Dr. Goldstein is a Michigan-based dentist who completed her General Practice Dental Residency at Michael Reese Hospital in Chicago. She has been in the private practice of general dentistry since 1990, with an emphasis on aesthetic dentistry. For more information, please visit www.berrisddspc.com or call 248-661-4000.

Melinda A. Hochgesang, DMD. Dr. Hochgesang is in private practice in Iowa. Known as "Dr. Mindy," she is a certified Invisalign provider and is proficient at root canals, removing teeth, and all other aspects of general dentistry. Known for her cheerful and friendly personality, Dr. Mindy is a regular guest on the *Paula Sands Live* TV show. To learn more about Dr. Mindy, visit www.byrumfamilydentistry.com.

Alina Krivitsky, DDS. Dr. Krivitsky specializes in the treatment of periodontal disease, soft and hard tissue augmentation, and dental implants. She is a diplomate of the American Board of Periodontology and an active member of the American Academy of Periodontology, the American Dental Association, and several other highly regarded organizations. To learn more about Dr. Krivitsky, visit www.implantperiocenter.com.

Renita Sansom, RDH. Dental Oncology Oral Hygiene Specialist at Dental Oncology Professionals of North Texas. For more information about Renita, visit www.dentaloncology.com.

Gregg Schneider, DDS. Dr. Schneider is a nutritional dentist practicing in New Jersey and a recognized expert in alternative medicine. Some of the maladies that he treats include sleep apnea, mouth sores due to chemotherapy, implant dentistry as well as cosmetic and family dentistry. Dr. Schneider's unique approach to dentistry has been profiled extensively in the media. To learn more about Dr. Schneider, visit www.drgreggschneider.com.

Harvey S. Shiffman, DDS. Dr. Shiffman is a graduate of Georgetown University School of Dentistry and specializes in laser systems, bringing new technology to the practice, which can offer numerous enhancements to standard procedures and many new and exciting options. Dr. Shiffman was recently awarded a fellowship in the Academy of Laser Dentistry and is personally involved in the use and development of cutting-edge technology. To learn more about Dr. Shiffman, visit www.boyntonlaserdental.com.

Michael Sinkin, DDS. Dr. Sinkin is a New York City–based dentist who has been in practice for over two decades. He owns a private general dental practice with emphasis on cosmetic and restorative dentistry. Dr. Sinkin is an active member in the American Dental Association, American Academy of Periodontology, Academy of General Dentistry, and a past president and member of the Board of Directors of NYU College of Dentistry Alumni Association. To learn more about Dr. Sinkin, visit www.michaelsinkindds.com.

HAIR

Jason Backe. Jason Backe is a colorist and president and CEO of ted gibson beauty. One of the most sought-after hair colorists in New York, Jason's clients include numerous models and actresses who love his color for its chic wearability. He was recently named celebrity colorist for L'Oreal Professionnel on the Color Advisory Board for the Colorist and is a part of Intercoiffure America/Canada Color Council. To learn more about Jason, visit www.tedgibsonbeauty.com.

Lola Bennett. Lola Bennett is a licensed hair stylist at the Yves Durif Salon at The Carlyle in New York. She specializes in treating women with hair loss and thinning, particularly through styling and scalp treatments.

Isaac Davidson. Isaac Davidson is an award-winning couture wig designer and hair stylist. He is the owner of WigBar in New York and counts among his clients fashion powerhouses Chanel and DKNY, as well as numerous celebrities. His work frequently appears on the runway and in top national publications. To learn more about Isaac, visit www.wigbar.com.

Lucinda Ellery. Lucinda Ellery is an internationally renowned hair replacement expert who has been helping women manage hair loss for over twenty-five years in the UK and Beverly Hills. Her passion and dedication to helping people with hair loss has resulted in a proactive approach to management options. Lucinda's work has appeared in numerous national publications in both the UK and United States. To learn more about Lucinda, visit www.lucindaellery-hairloss.com.

Barry Hendrickson. Barry Hendrickson is owner of the famed wig salon Bitz-n-Pieces in Manhattan. Known for his commitment to helping women feel like themselves during cancer treatment with an array of natural-looking wigs and services by top-notch stylists, Barry shares his secrets for hair and makeup in his book *Looking Like You: A Step-by-Step Guide for Medical Hair Replacement*. To learn more about Barry, visit www.bitzandpieces.com.

Lisa Lewis. Lisa is a young cancer survivor and the founder of Wig It2 in Clovis, California. While in treatment, Lisa realized the need for empathy, creativity, knowledge and coverage options for a young woman like herself. She combined wig and salon services like extensions and hair bonding to help women in treatment discreetly and with respect. To learn more about Lisa, visit www.wigit2.com

Toni Love. Toni Love is an international hair expert, platform stylist, and educator. She is a twice-published author and currently owns Toni Love's Training Center in Atlanta, Georgia. Her book, *The World of Wigs, Weaves and Extensions*, is a must-have for all successful stylists using artificial hair. To learn more about Toni, visit www.tonilove.com.

Helen Owens. An alopecia areata survivor, Helen Owens has spent decades transforming women suffering from hair thinning into women with hair they love. She has garnered numerous awards for her work, including being named a finalist in the race for the Bay Area's Most Influential African-Americans, and appears frequently in print and the media. To learn more about Ms. Owens, please visit www.hersecrethairextensions.com.

Isaac Mann. Isaac Mann is a Boca Raton and Boston-based hair guru who has appeared in numerous fashion publications alongside his partner, international makeup artist Tim Quinn.

Corey Powell. Corey Powell is a world-renowned hair designer and colorist known for his famously blond celebrity clients and fashion icons. He has been featured as an expert in many top print publications. Today Corey can be found at the Sally Hershberger Salon in Los Angeles. To learn more about Corey, visit www.coreypowellhair.com.

MAKEUP ARTISTS

Courtney Akai. Courtney Akai is a makeup artist and eyelash extension artisan whose work is consistently featured in top media publications and on celebrities. A pioneer of the craft in New York City, Courtney is owner of the Courtney Akai Lash Boutique in New York City. To learn more about Courtney, visit www.courtneyakai.com.

Cindy Barbakov. Cindy Barbakov is a New York City makeup artist who has done campaigns for major designers and fashion publications with her company, CYN Production. Her work has appeared everywhere from the red carpet to elaborate music videos and editorial spreads. To learn more about Cindy, visit www.cynproduction.com.

Andrea Charles. Andrea Charles is a New York City makeup artist and creator of City Girl Beauty Project, a not-for-profit organization empowering survivors of domestic violence and human trafficking. She started her career in NYC, enhancing the faces of numerous entertainment personalities. To learn more about Andrea and her inspiring philanthropic efforts, visit www.andreadcharles.com.

Krista Embry. Krista Embry is a celebrity makeup artist, model, and consultant. She is the creator of "Live Love Life," a DVD devoted to helping women face the day with confidence during cancer treatment. Krista has worked with countless celebrities, musicians, sports icons, and politicians, including a US president and vice president. To learn more about Krista, visit www.kristaembry.com.

Ramy Gafni. Ramy Gafni is an internationally known makeup artist and author of *Ramy Gafni's Beauty Therapy: The Ultimate Guide to Looking and Feeling Great While Living with Cancer.* Ever in demand for his makeup artistry and eyebrow shaping, Ramy continues to see clients while overseeing the development of the RAMY beauty therapy product collection. He has appeared in the pages of every major fashion and beauty magazine and on many national television shows. To learn more about Ramy, visit www.ramy.com.

Dee Dee Jones-McCuen. Dee Dee Jones-McCuen is a makeup artist, model, and founder of Posh Pout. Dee Dee is known for her attention to detail, creating faces with perfect brows, fresh skin, glamorous lashes, and a perfect lip. She has worked with numerous celebrities and for television. To learn more about Dee Dee, visit www.posh-pout.com.

Fawn Monique. Fawn Monique is a celebrity makeup artist known for her looks at New York Fashion Week and on numerous film stars. She is also founder of BeYouFirst, an organization that helps underprivileged individuals discover his or her beauty, inside and out. She also strives to make a difference in the beauty industry by teaching fellow artists to connect inner and outer beauty with healthy eco-conscious-aligned cosmetics. To learn more about Fawn, visit www.fawnmonique.com.

Tim Quinn. Tim Quinn is a celebrity makeup artist and National Director of Creative Artistry for Giorgio Armani Beauty. As the US front man for Giorgio Armani Beauty, Tim has been featured as one of the "25 Beauty Stars" in *W* magazine and won a 2011 Genius Award in *Elle* magazine as a Genius Makeup Artist, among many other awards. To learn more about Tim, visit www.giorgioarmanibeauty-usa.com.

MEDICAL TATTOO ARTISTS

Cathi Locati. Cathi Locati is an areola architect known for her incredible 3-D photorealistic nipple repigmentation. She works with numerous plastic surgeons in the metropolitan New York area, who admire her work to recreate natural, beautiful nipples. She is also the creator of 7th Dimension Illusion Breastmounds, which mimic the look of the whole breast on mastectomy patients. To learn more about Cathi, visit www.cathilocatico.com.

Julie Michaud. Julie Michaud is a Boston-based makeup artist specializing in permanent cosmetics, micropigmentation, areola repigmentation, and scar camouflage. After working with numerous celebrities, Julie opened her salon, Prettyology, in 1998, where she and her team offer cosmetic skin treatments, permanent makeup, and other aesthetic services. To learn more about Julie, visit www.prettyology.com.

Laura Reed, OD, CPCP, FAAM. Dr. Reed is a paramedical tattoo artist and licensed optometric physician. She is board-certified in permanent cosmetics and specializes in medical micropigmentation techniques such as scar reduction, reconstructive camouflage, and areola repigmentation. She is a multiple winner of "Best in the West" awards. To learn more about Dr. Reed, visit www.artisticcosmeticsolutions.com.

BREAST SURGEON

JOHN A. RIMMER, MD. DR. RIMMER is board-certified by the American Board of Surgery and a fellow of both the Royal College of Surgeons,

England, and the Royal College of Surgeons, Edinburgh, Scotland. He is currently a member of the American Society of Breast Surgeons and is the medical director of the Kristin Hoke Breast Health Program at Jupiter Medical Center. To learn more about Dr. Rimmer, visit www.johnrimmermd.com.

PLASTIC SURGEONS

Alan J. Bauman, MD. Dr. Bauman is a board-certified plastic surgeon and founder and medical director of Bauman Medical Group. He is one of only approximately one hundred board-certified hair restoration physicians in the world. He has built an international practice, treated nearly fifteen thousand hair loss patients since 1997, and has been extensively featured in the world's leading media in print, radio, and television as a medical expert and successful early adopter of the most advanced technologies in the treatment of hair loss. To learn more about Dr. Bauman, visit www.baumanmedical. com.

Danielle Deluca-Pytell, MD. Dr. DeLuca-Pytell is a board-certified plastic surgeon specializing in breast and body contouring, facial cosmetic surgery, breast reconstruction, cosmetic surgery after weight loss, and hair transplantation. She has published multiple articles in surgical journals such as *Plastic and Reconstructive Surgery* and the textbook *Breast Augmentation*. Due to her extensive research and expertise, she has lectured at national scientific meetings for aesthetic surgery. To learn more about Dr. Deluca-Pytell, visit www. delucapytell.com.

Melissa Doft, MD. Dr. Doft is a board-certified plastic surgeon and assistant professor of surgery at Weill Cornell Medical College at New York–Presbyterian Hospital. She has studied aspects of breast surgery both from the oncological side as a general surgeon and the reconstructive side as a plastic surgeon. Her areas of expertise include breast surgery and breast reconstruction, facial reconstruction surgery, and burn and wound correction. To learn more about Dr. Doft, visit www.doftplasticsurgery.com.

Larry Fan, MD. Dr. Fan is a board-certified plastic surgeon, voted one of America's Top Plastic Surgeons for the past five years by the Consumers Research Council of America. He is founding director of 77 Plastic Surgery. He is also an accomplished scientist and has received several national awards for his research in plastic surgery. To learn more about Dr. Fan, visit www.77plasticsurgery.com.

Allen Gabriel, MD, FACS. Dr. Gabriel is a board-certified plastic and reconstructive surgeon and founder of the Pink Lemonade Project, which educates and supports those affected by breast cancer. Currently he is the associate professor of surgery at Loma Linda University Medical Center and in private practice in Vancouver, Washington. He has authored more than ten dozen abstracts, manuscripts, and book chapters and continues to share his knowledge both nationally and internationally. To learn more about Dr. Gabriel, visit www.swplasticsurg.com.

James Marotta, MD. Dr. Marotta is a dual board-certified facial plastic surgeon with particular expertise and interest in minimally invasive (endoscopic) facial plastic surgery, facial rejuvenation, and hair restoration. He is Clinical Assistant Professor of Surgery at SUNY Stony Brook and a fellow of the American Academy of Facial Plastic and Reconstructive Surgery (AAFPRS). To learn more about Dr. Marotta, visit www.marottamd.com.

Ariel N. Rad, MD, PhD. Dr. Rad is a board-certified plastic surgeon and assistant professor and director of Aesthetic Plastic Surgery in the Department of Plastic Surgery at Johns Hopkins. While at Johns Hopkins, Dr. Rad and his colleagues pioneered the most advanced microsurgical techniques in breast reconstruction, such as the landmark publication describing the "LSGAP flap." He is also in private practice in Washington, DC. To learn more about Dr. Rad, visit www.sherberandrad.com.

C. Andrew Salzberg, MD. Dr. Salzberg is a New York board-certified plastic surgeon who specializes in cosmetic surgery and breast surgery, including breast reconstruction. He is the chief of plastic surgery at St. John's Riverside Hospital - Dobbs Ferry Pavilion, and Westchester Medical Center. Dr. Salzberg is best known as the pioneer of Direct to Implant and AlloDerm Breast Reconstruction. To learn more about Dr. Salzberg, visit www.nygplasticsurgery.com.

SKIN CARE

Kimberly Luker. Kimberly Luker is the creator of the natural, nourishing skin care line Botanicals for Hope, which she developed after being diagnosed with an aggressive form of stage IIB breast cancer. Kimberly's clients range from those who have always had dry or sensitive skin to those whose skin issues began as the result of medications, and her products are gaining popularity with oncologists and cancer patients alike. To learn more about Kimberly, visit www.botanicalsforhope.com.

Kristin Provvidenti. Kristin Provvidenti is a paramedical makeup artist and cancer survivor. She is the creator of Stella Bella Mineral Cosmetics, a botanically based, bismuth-free line of cosmeceutical skin-care products developed for highly sensitive skin particularly experienced during chemotherapy. Stella Bella has received awards and been featured in many national publications. For more information about Kristin, visit www.mystellabellashop.com.

Anne C. Willis, LE. Anne C. Willis is the founder of De La Terre skin care and director of Oncology Skin Therapeutics, bringing over thirty years of experience and knowledge to a new generation of skin therapists. As a pioneer in medical skin therapies, Ms. Willis developed some of the first skin-care programs designed specifically for pre- and postoperative skin therapy. Ms. Willis lectures nationally regarding holistic skin therapies, collaborative care for medical institutions, and skin reactions incurred by patients receiving combined chemotherapy. To learn more about Ms. Willis, visit counterrevolutionary.

Jennifer Young. Jennifer Young is microbiologist and the creator of Defiant Beauty, skin care and beauty collections formulated for use by those going through treatment for cancer. She is an associate member of the Royal Society of Medicine and a lecturer in nutrition, skin care, and product formulation. Jennifer is also the editor of Beauty Despite Cancer, the website of Defiant Beauty. To learn more about Jennifer, visit www.beautydespitecancer.co.uk.

STYLE

Jennifer Manghisi. Jennifer Manghisi is a New York City–based style expert and author of *A Sarcastic Guide to Beating Breast Cancer*, published in October 2012. In it, she shares what she learned on her journey to survival of stage 0 noninvasive breast cancer. She is now at work on her second book while working at EmblemHealth. To learn more about Jennifer, visit www.jmanghisi.com.

Colin Megaro. Colin Megaro is a NYC/LA-based celebrity wardrobe stylist and fashion expert who has done work for print and television, including personal appearances on several notable shows. His signature look combines the glamor of old Hollywood with the timelessness of classic, wearable pieces. A three-time cancer survivor himself, Colin is actively involved with the American Cancer Society GLAAD and Jeffrey Fashion Cares. To learn more about Colin, visit www.colinmegaro.com.

Elizabeth Thompson, MD. Dr. Thompson is radiation oncologist and reconstructive surgeon. After years of breast surveillance, biopsies, and endless consultations with genetic counselors, Dr. Thompson underwent prophylactic mastectomies. The experience of recovering from this surgery and the interactions with her physicians led her to begin working in the reconstructive surgery practice, helping other women with the difficult decision-making regarding and recovery from breast surgery. She is also the creator of BFFL Co, a fashionable line of bags, bras, and surgical accessories to provide comfort and convenience in the modern day of breast treatment. To learn more about Dr. Thomson, visit www.bfflco.com.

FITNESS

Marsha Danzig, MEd. Marsha Danzig is a yoga instructor, RYT 500, movement therapist, and life coach. She is a childhood cancer survivor and the founder of Color Me Yoga, a therapeutic program for children, and Yoga for Amputees. Marsha is also the author of *Fierce Joy*, a memoir about how to maintain joy, no matter what. To learn more about Marsha, visit www.fiercejoy.net.

Lockey Maisonneuve. Lockey Maisonneuve is a certified Cancer Exercise Specialist, breast cancer survivor, and founder of MovingOn, a rehabilitative exercise program for breast cancer patients. She is on the Community Advisory Board for the Carol G. Simon Cancer Center at Overlook Hospital and has been featured in national print and other media outlets. To learn about Lockey, visit www.lockeymaisonneuve.com.

Carol Michaels. Carol Michaels is the founder and creator of Recovery Fitness, an exercise program designed to help cancer patients recover from surgery and treatments. The author of *Exercises for Cancer Survivors*, Carol is a Cancer Exercise Specialist and consultant and has been a fitness professional for more than eighteen years. To learn more about Carol, visit www.carolmichaelsfitness.com.

WELLNESS

Magali Chohan, PhD. Dr. Magali Chohan is a lecturer in nutrition at the School of Life Sciences in Kingston University and a registered nutritionist. She holds diplomas in aromatherapy, herbal medicine, and nutritional medicine, followed by a PhD in nutrition. Dr. Chohan is a member of the Nutrition Society and the British Herbal Medicine Association, researching bioactive compounds in foods with a focus on polyphenols in culinary herbs and spices. To learn more about Dr. Chohan, email magalichohan@hotmail.co.uk.

Kristy Fishman. Kristy Fishman is an insurance agent and breast cancer survivor with extensive knowledge in many aspects of health insurance policies, procedures, and laws and patient advocacy. She is also an active participant in several breast cancer clinical trial study groups with UCLA and counsels individuals who have been diagnosed with breast cancer. To learn more about Kristy, visit www.FishmanBenefits.com.

Jodie Guerrero. Jodie Guerrero is a Queensland-based consumer advocate, activist, and creator of Jodie's Journey, chronicling her incredible battle with incurable follicular non-Hodgkin's lymphoma. Her story has been featured in numerous Australian media outlets, and she is a fierce advocate for women's health and cancer research. To learn more about Jodie, visit www.jodiesjourney.com.

Elena Klimenko, MD. Dr. Klimenko is a board-certified internist and licensed in medical acupuncture and homeopathy. She uses a blend of Western and alternative medicines to give clients well-rounded, integrative treatment solutions. She is currently an active teaching faculty member at the Center for Education of Doctors in Homeopathy, and she is certified in noninvasive cosmetic procedures such as Botox and fillers injections. To learn more about Dr. Klimenko, visit www.drelenaklimenko.com.

April Dawn Ricchuito, MSW. Ms. Ricchuito is a young cancer survivor, writer, speaker, consultant, and health-care advocate who brings a unique voice to the field of health and wellness by combining traditional evidence-based techniques with ancient practices such as yoga and newer findings in contemplative sciences. Ms. Ricchuito has been recognized as a part of "Generation Inspiration" and is named as one of 20 Young Champions for Women by the White Ribbon Alliance and WIE Symposium, presented by Donna Karan and Arianna Huffington. To learn more about Ms. Ricchuito, visit www.verbalvandalism.com.

EMOTIONAL SUPPORT

Jennifer Alhasa. Jennifer Alhasa is a cancer coach and therapist. A breast cancer survivor, Jennifer has dedicated herself to developing and teaching her own advanced approach to transformation through energy healing and intuitive life coaching. She has worked one-on-one with patients at Memorial Sloan-Kettering Cancer Center in New York and other institutions. To learn more about Jennifer, visit www.about.me/jenniferalhasa.

Leslie Davenport. Leslie Davenport is an author, psychotherapist, and founding member of one of the nation's largest integrative medicine centers associated with a hospital, the Institute for Health & Healing at California Pacific Medical Center in San Francisco. For the last twenty years, she has guided thousands of people to harness the source of healing within using the ancient tool of guided imagery. Because the efficacy of imagery is now backed by years of research, she has established guided imagery programs in five hospitals and has recently published a book, *Healing and Transformation through Self-Guided Imagery*. To learn more about Leslie, visit www.lesliedavenport.com.

Melanie Greenberg, PhD. Dr. Greenberg is a clinical health psychologist in Marin County, California, a former Professor and expert on mind-body issues for *Psychology Today*. She is author of *The Stress-Resistant Brain*, to be published in 2016 by New Harbinger. To learn more about Dr. Greenberg, please visit www.melaniegreenbergphd.com.

Elyn Jacobs. Elyn Jacobs is a professional cancer strategist and the executive director for the Emerald Heart Cancer Foundation. A breast cancer survivor herself, she mentors women who are coping with issues of well-being associated with breast cancer and its aftermath. To learn more about Elyn, visit www.elynjacobs.com.

Samantha Keen. Samantha is a therapist and consultant at VitalSwitch, New York. Having used the techniques of ISIS to recover from chronic fatigue syndrome herself, Samantha has a special insights into vitality issues, including chronic fatigue and burnout, as well as how to manage energy to increase personal performance. To learn more about Samantha, visit www. vitalswitch.com.

Matteus Levell. Matteus is a meditation expert and therapist and the founder of VitalSwitch, a New York–based Wellness Consultancy that specializes in teaching meditation-based skills for use in daily life. Matteus has over twenty years of experience and training in meditation and Inner Space Techniques (IST), which incorporates a practical and effective guided meditation practice with a gentle but deep emotional exploration. To learn more about Matteus, visit www.vitalswitch.com.

Gary R. McClain, PhD. Dr. McClain is a patient advocate, therapist, and author who specializes in working with clients who are facing chronic and catastrophic medical diagnoses, as well as their caregivers and health-care professionals. He has authored books on body-mind-spirit topics, as well as a supplementary textbook for nursing and allied health-care programs, *After the Diagnosis: How Patients React and How to Help Them Cope* (Cengage/ Delmar, 2010). He has published articles for numerous health-related publications. His website, www.JustGotDiagnosed.com, provides information and inspiration for individuals living with chronic illness, caregivers, and professionals. To learn more about Dr. McClain, visit www.JustGotDiagnosed. com.

Some Chemotherapy Side Effects on Skin

Please note: This list is not exhaustive, and only chemotherapy drugs available at the time of writing and which have documented side effects are noted. See your doctor for information about side effects for those which are not listed.

Class of Drug and General Side Effects	Drug/Brand Name	Skin Side Effects
Alkylating Agents: redness; peeling, darkening in skin folds	Cyclophosphamide (Cytoxan)	Bruising/bleeding; rash; change of color to skin; change in nail texture; darkening of skin folds and sometimes mouth; redness; peeling
	Cisplatin (Platinol)	Rash; itchiness; Raynaud's phenomenon (discoloration to fingers or toes); flushing; darkening of nails
	Vinblastine (Velban)	Increased sensitivity to sunlight; Hand-Foot Syndrome.
	Temozolomide (Temodor)	Xerosis (dryness, scaly, itch, and redness); rash
	Procarbazine (Matulane)	Darkening of skin folds and sometimes mouth.
	Oxaliplatin (Eloxatin)	Hand-Foot Syndrome
	Vindesine (Eldisine)	Inflammation at site drip; rash
	Lomustine (CeeNU)	Rash; bruising; pallor; red spots
	Melphalan (Alkeran)	Rash; pale/yellowed skin; itchiness

	Drug	Side effects
	Carmustine (BiCNU, Carustine)	Pale or darkened skin
	Busulfan (Myerlan, Busulfex IV)	Swelling; rash; itchy dry skin; hyperpigmentation
	Hexamethylmelamine (Hexalen)	Peripheral Neuropathy
Antimetabolites: Skin swelling; sensitivity to sun; flushing; itchiness; nail discoloration or malformation	5-FU (Adrucil)	Dry, cracking and/or peeling skin; nail and tooth discoloration; increased sensitivity to sunlight; Hand-Foot syndrome
	Methotrexate (Amethopterin, Floex, Mexate, MTXRheumatrex, Trexall)	Photosensitivity; recall reactions (rash); Eccrine squamous metaplasia (very rare: red plaques or a papular, crusted eruption at injection site)
	Capecitabine (Xeloda)	Hand-Foot Syndrome
	Hydroxyurea (Hydrea, Droxia)	Rash; skin ulceration; inflammation; peripheral and facial redness; hyperpigmentation; dry and fragile skin and nails; scaling; darkening of skin folds and sometimes mouth
	Cladribine (Leustatin)	Swelling
	Cytarabine (Cytosar-U, Tarabine)	Rash
	Gemcitabine (Gemzar)	Rash; injection site reactions
	Cladribine (Leustatin)	Swelling
	Raltitrexed (Tomudex, TDX, ZD 1964)	Rash, itchiness

	Mercaptopurine (Purinethol)	Yellowed skin
Antineoplastic Agents/Anti-tumor Antiobiotics: Hand-Foot syndrome; nail separation; sun damage; hyperpigmentation	Epirubicin hydrochloride (Ellence)	Darkening of skin; mild rash or itching
	Mitoxantrone (Novatrone)	Pale skin; bruising
	Mitomycin (Mutamycin, Mitomycin-C)	Rashes; swelling at the injection site; mouth inflammation. The most important dermatological problem with this drug, however, is the dying of tissue and consequent sloughing off of tissue which results if the drug is extravasated (leaked) during injection. Leaking may occur with or without an accompanying stinging or burning sensation and even if there is adequate blood return when the injection needle is aspirated. There have been reports of delayed erythea (redness) and/or ulceration occurring either at or distant from the injection site, weeks to months after Mitomycin.
	Dactinomycin (Cosmegen)	Red spots
	Mitoxantrone (Onkotrone, Novatrone)	Mouth inflammation; bluish-discoloration of eye whites; leaking at the infusion site resulting in redness, swelling, pain, burning, necrosis and/or blue discoloration of the skin

	Doxorubicin (Adriamycin, Myocet, Doxil, Caelyx)	Subacute cutaneous lupus erythematosus (SCLE, a sun-sensitive rash); darkening of skin folds and sometimes mouth; darkening of nail beds; Hand-Foot Syndrome; sun damage
	Daunorubicin	Radiation Recall (tissue damage from prior radiation can become redder)
	Bleomycin (Blenoxane)	Darkening of skin folds and sometimes mouth; Hand-Foot Syndrome
Mitotic Inhibitors/Plant Alkaloids/Taxanes: Hand-Foot Syndrome; itchiness/peeling; swelling; nail malformation or abnormalities	Paclitaxel (Abraxane, Taxol)	Shedding nails; redness or dryness of the skin; itching; neutrophilic eccrine hidradenitis ("Sweet's Syndrome" characterized by red bumps, see your dermatologist); neuropathy (numbness/tingling in fingers/toes); Hand-Foot Syndrome
	Docetaxel (Taxotere)	Redness or dryness; "Sweet's Syndrome" (characterized by red bumps, see your dermatologist); Hand-Foot Syndrome; scleroderma (hardening of the skin); nail changes
	Vincristine (Oncovin)	Peeling; swelling; nail abnormalities
Corticosteroids	Prednisone (Delasone, Liquid Pred, Meticorten, Orasone, Predicin-M, Predinicot, Sterapred, Sterapred DS)	Bruising; fungal infections; rash

Category	Drug	Side effects
Glucocorticoid Steroid	Dexamethasone (Decadron)	Acne
Aromatose Inhibitors (Hormone Therapy): Red nodules under skin; sun-sensitive rash; rashes	Exemestane (Aromasin)	Swelling of mouth/lips; rash; blushing; hot flashes; redness; hair growth
	Anastrozole (Arimidex)	
Hormones/SERMs (Selective Estrogen-Receptor Modulators)	Tamoxifen (Nolvadex, Zoladex, Lupron)	Hot flashes; infection; loss of elasticity; increased wrinkling; severe dryness; hair thinning and partial alopecia; acneiform rash; photosensitivity; bruising; irritation; skin thinning which makes skin prone to spitting and/or an aged appearance. On rare occasions, urticaria, a rare allergic reaction resulting in skin rash and welts, as reported in *The World Journal of Surgical Oncology* [2007]
Monoclonal antibodies	Bevacizumab (Avastin)	Dry skin; slow wound healing; inflammation of skin
	Rituximab (Rituxan)	Redness
	Trastuzumab (Herceptin)	Nail changes; rash/hives; itchy skin; swelling of mouth and lips
EGFR inhibitors	Cetuximab (Erbitux)	Acne

Category	Drug	Side effects
a. **Tyrosine-kinase Inhibitor:** infections around fingernail and toenails; hair changes; skin fissures in hands and feet; pigmentation changes	Erlotinib (Tarceva)	Peeling; flaking; acne; inflammation of hair follicles/pimples; inflamed areas around nails; facial hair growth and redness
	Gefitinib (Iressa)	Dry skin; itchy skin; blisters on hands and feet; inflammation of hair follicles/pimples; inflammation/infection around nails; facial hair growth; facial redness
b. **Proteasome inhibitor**	Bortezomib (Velcade)	Rash
c. **Trotease inhibitor**	Indinavir (Crixivan)	Rash; itchiness; scaling; dry skin; and leukocytoclastic vasculitis (purpling of skin); rash (including Stevens-Johnson syndrome and itchiness/skin lesions); nail and skin hyperpigmentation; ingrown toenails and/or inflammation around nails
d. **Topoisomerase inhibitors:** Infections around finger and toe nails; skin cracking in hands and feet; pigmentation changes	Etoposide (Eposin, Etopophos, Vepesid)	Rash; inflammation at drip site; signs of allergic reaction (flushing, swelling of lips, tongue and face)

e. PARP (Poly [ADP-ribose] polymerase) Inhibitors	AZD2281 (Olaparib)		Rash; itchiness; scaliness
Targeted Therapy	Imantib (Gleevac)		Canker sores; rash; petechia (broken blood vessels); dryness; itchiness; periorbital edema (inflammation around the eye); peeling skin; psoriasis; skin lesions; nail disorders; skin pigmentation changes; photosensitivity and purpura (purple discoloration)
Cytokines	IL-2 (Interleukon-2)		Itchiness; Hand-Foot Syndrome
	IFN-x		Rash
	L-4		Flushing

Skin Treatments Suggested by Experts
Please note: Always check in with your doctor before trying any new treatments.

Skin Treatment	Hi-tech, Specialized and Pharmaceutical	Drugstore	Natural	
Facial Dry skin cleanser	Skinceuticals Gentle Cleanser	Vanicream Cleansing Bar	Calm Skin Arnica Mask by Eminence	
	VIVITÉ® Daily Facial Cleanser	Cetaphil Gentle Skin Cleanser	Dr. Hauschka Cleansing Cream	
	EvoSkin Hydrating Skin Cleanser	CeraVe Hydrating Cleanser	Nature's Gate Purifying Liquid Soap	
	Lindi Face Wash	Neutrogena Extra Gentle Cleanser	Yogurt Mask (see appendix)	
		Dove Sensitive Skin Unscented Beauty Bar	Monica Hall Spa Cleansing Milk	
		La Roche-Posay Toleriane Dermo-Cleanser	Stella Bella Pure Actives Dermacalm Cleanser for Dry, Sensitive and Medically Compromised Skin	
		Vichy Pureté Thermale 3-in-1 Calming Cleansing Solution	Botanicals for Hope Soapless Facial Cleanser	

Facial Moisturizer (skin dry, needs oil)			
	Dr. Brandt Crème de LUXE	Aquaphor Healing Ointment	Rescue Wounded Skincare system, de la Terre Skincare (www.delaterre.com)
	Crème de la Mer	Avène Extreme Tolerance Cream	Monica Hall Spa Daytime Elixir
	Gel de la Mer	Cetaphil Moisturizing Cream	Natura Health Products Skin Protect
	Cosmedix Mystic Moisture Mist	Aveeno Ultra-Calming Daily Moisturizer with SPF 15	Dr. Hauschka's Rose Cream
	Skinceuticals Hydrating B5 Gel	Eucerin Everyday Protection SPF 30 Face Lotion	Jojoba Oil
	Skinceuticals Emollience	CeraVe Facial Moisturizing Lotion Cream (both AM and PM formulas)	Pure shea butter
	Neocutis Journee Bio-restorative Day Cream with PSP SPF 30+	Vanicream Moisturizing Skin Care Cream	Extra virgin coconut or olive oil
	VIVITÉ® Daily Antioxidant Facial Serum		Zoe Organics Extreme Cream
	AVA MD Extreme Specialist Face Cream		Zoe Organics Love My Body Oil

	Linacare Transforming Face Cream	Avocado Oil
	Hylatopic Plus (Rx)	Argon Oil
	Epiceram (Rx)	
	Lindi Face Moisturizer	
	Lindi Face Serum	
	Actifirm Renovation Cream	
Facial Hydration (skin may be oily but needs moisture)	SkinCeuticals Hydrating B5 Gel	Monica Hall Spa Cell-Lift Ageless Serum
	Skinceuticals Phyto Corrective Gel	Botanicals for Hope Bioactive Serum
	PCA Skin Collagen Hydrator	
Eye Cream	Replenix Eye Repair Cream (note: contains retinol and may not be suitable for all skin)	Indie Lee Eye Balm
	Neocutis Bio-restorative Eye Cream with PSP	
	Lindi Eye Hydrator	

Hydrating Mists (for use during the day to replenish moisture)	AVA MD Antioxidant Mist	Cosmedix Mystic Moisture Mist	Avène Thermal Spring Water	Milk Spritz (see appendix)	De La Terre Skincare Supports Healthy Skin Herb Rich Mist
Body Soap/Wash	L'Occitane Shea Butter Extra Gentle Soap	Lindi Body Wash	Dove Cream Oil Body Wash	CeraVe Hydrating Cleanser	Neutrogena Rainbath Deep Moisture Body Wash
	Dove Sensitive Skin Unscented Beauty Bar	Aveeno Moisturizing Daily Body Wash	Burt's Bees Baby Bee Nourishing Body Oil	Dr. Bronners	Whole Food's 365 Brand glycerin bar
	Epsom salts or Dead Sea Salts with Lavender Oil	Indie Lee Cleansing Bar	Celebrating Pink Moisturizing Body Bar		

Body Moisturizer			Lindi Body Wash
	Kiehl's Crème de Corps	Cetaphil Moisturizing Cream	-
	Actifirm Decollete Firm	Eucerin Plus Intensive Repair Lotion	Spectrum Organic Coconut Oil
	Actifirm Neck Firm Cream	Neutrogena Body Oil	Vitamin E Oil
	Kiehl's Argon Body Lotion	Body Shop Body Butter	Clearly Natural Glycerin Body Lotion (unscented)
	Origins Body Butter	Aveeno Daily Moisturizing Lotion	Simplers Organic Lavender Essential Oil
	Linacare Rehydrating Body Cream	Lubriderm Bath Oil	Burt's Bees Nourishing Body Oil
	Linacare Body Cream Daily Moisture	CeraVe Moisturizing Cream	SkinFree Super Moisture Body Balm
	Ahava Dermud Nourishing Body Cream	Aveeno Skin Relief Moisturizing Cream	Celebrating Pink Pure Unscented Buttercream Lotion
	Lindi Body Lotion	La Roche-Posay Toleriane Body Lotion	zoa organics extreme cream
		Vaseline Body Lption with Vitamin E and Aloe Vera	Botanicals for Hope Olive & Aloe Body Lotion

Body Exfoliation	Sugar Exfoliation (see appendix)		
	Pangea Organics Scrub		
	Indie Lee The Body Scrub		
Hand Soap	Clearly Natural Liquid Glycerin Hand Soap		
	Avalon Organics Glycerin Hand Soap		
	Dr. Bronner Organic Hand Soap		
	Pangea Organic Hand Soap		
Itchiness/irritation/exema:	De La Terre Skin Care Comforts Inflamed Skin System	Sarna Original Anti-Itch Lotion	Pramosone or Pramagel (antineuralgia preparation, Rx)
	Burt's Bees Baby Bee Nourishing Body Oil	CeraVe Moisturizing Cream	Elidel Cream (non-steroid, Rx)

	Steroid cream (Rx)	OTC 1% hydrocortisone cream	Hibiscus Calendula Recovery Masque by Eminence
	Anti-Irritant Laser Relief, Dr. Brandt	VaniCream Moisturizing Skin Cream	Bag Balm (for hands)
	Dapsone (anti-inflammatory, Rx)		Indie Lee The Body Balm
	La Roche-Posay Toleriane Cleanser (cleanser)		De La Terre Skin Care Mineral Rich Salt
	Actifirm Active Skin Soother		
	Lindi Face Serum		
	Lindi Soothing Balm		
Redness	Skinceuticals Phyto Corrective Gel	(see products below for rosacea)	Eminence Calm Skin Arnica Mask
	Neocutis Peche Redness Control Serum		
	Clinique Redness Solutions Line		
Loss of Elasticity/Aging Appearance	Mild dermabrasion (see doctor)	Clarisonic Classic Sonic Skin Cleansing System	Monica Hall Spa The Organic Face Lift

	Skinceuticals LHA Cleansing Gel	Mild OTC retinol cream	Cornmeal Mask (see appendix)
	Oxygen facials (see doctor)		
	Crease Release, Dr. Brandt		
	Atralin (Rx)		
	SkinMedica TNS Essential Serum		
	Skinceuticals Phloretin-CF with PSP		
Dark Spots/Hyperpigmentation	Hydroquinine 4.0% (Rx)	Natura Skin Protect	
	Prescription retinoids (not for all skin types, see your doctor)		
	Skinceuticals C E Ferulic		
	Dr. Brandt Flaws No More		
	Neocutis Skin Lightening Cream		
Rosacea cleanser	Skin Effects Redness Control Calming Cleanser	Cetaphil Gentle Skin Cleanser	Eminence Calm Skin Arnica Mask

Rosacea treatment	Clinique Redness Solutions Line	La Roche-Posay Toleriane Dermo-Cleanser	Eminence Quince and Ice Wine Mask / White Clay Mask (see appendix)
	Topical sulfur agents (ask your doctor)	Olay Definity Corrective Protective Lotion withSPF 15	
	Lindi Skin Facial Serum	Eucerin Q10 Redness Relief Anti-Aging Serum	
	Dr. Brandt Pore Effect	Aveeno Active Naturals Ultra-Calming Daily Moisturizer SPF 15	
	(Rx) Metrogel and Finacea	Lubriderm Seriously Sensitive Lotion for Extra Sensitive Dry Skin	
	Clinique Redness Solutions Line	La Roche-Posay Rosaliac Anti-Redness Moisturizer	
	Skin Effects Redness Control Laser Correcting Treatment		
	Skin Effects Redness Control Daily Moisturizer SPF 30+		
Acne - cleanser	Sudamane	Avène Cleanance Gel Cleanser	Burts Bees Natural Acne Solutions Purifying Gel Cleanser

Acne Treatment - Prescription	Skinceuticals LHA Cleansing Gel
	Calming Zinc bar soap
	NeoStrata Antibacterial Facial Cleanser
	Aczone gel (Rx)
	Atralin gel. 05% (Rx)
	Finacea gel or Azelex (Rx)
	Veltin (Rx)
	Cleocin (Rx)
	Clindamicin (Rx)
	Low-dose antibiotics (Rx)
	Dapsone(Rx)
	topical sulfur agent (ask your doctor)
	Herb Rich Clay Purifies Blemished Skin, De La Terre Skincare
Acne Treatment - over the counter	Blemishes No More, Dr. Brandt
	mild benzoyl peroxide if skin tolerates it (2.5%)
	Pure Aloe Vera

Pores No More, Dr. Brandt	low-strength salicylic acid	Burt's Bees Blemish Stick
Skinceuticals Phyto Corrective Gel		
Sunscreen - Face		California Baby Face anjd Body Sunscreen SPF 30
Anthelios SPF 30	Neutrogena Age Shield Face Sunblock	Alba Botanica Green Tea Sunblock SPF 45
Skinceuticals Sheer UV Defense SPF 50 (tinted)	Aveeno Ultra-Calming Daily Moisturizer SPF 30	Alba Botanica Very Emollient Sunblock with Lavender SPF 45
Neocutis Journee Bio-restorative Day Cream with PSP SPF 30+		
Alyria Multi Age Correction SPF 15		
SolRX Dry Zinc SPF 40		
Kiehl's Super Fluid UV Defense 50+		
Elta MD Skincare UV Physical Sunblock SPF 41		
Vivite Daily Facial Moisturizer with SPF 30		
Radx 8 Hour Waterproof Sunblock		

	LindiSkin Sunblock		
Sunscreen - Body	Solbar SPF 50	Neutrogena Fresh Cooling Sunblock Gel SPF 45	Soleo Organics All Natural Sunscreen SPF 30
	EltaMD Skincare UV Physical SPF 41	Eucerin Everyday Protection Body Lotion SPF 15	California Baby Face and Body Sunscreen SPF 30
	Total Block Clear SPF 65		Botanicals for Hope Daily Sun Defense Cream, SPF 30
Lips	L'Occitane Shea Butter Lip Balm Stick	Aquaphor	Zoe Organics Refresh Lip Balm
	PCA Skin Peptide Lip Therapy	Aveeno Essential Moisture Lip Conditioner with SPF 15	Celebrating Pink Lip Balm
	Lindi Lip Balm	Aveeno Intense Relief Medicated Lip Therapy	Alba Un-Petroleum Jelly
	Lindi Face Serum	La Roche-Posay Ceralip	Dr. Bronner Organic Lip Balm
	Carrington RadiaCare Lip Balm		Pure Coconut Oil
			Pure Shea Butter
			Pure Aloe Vera

Skin Cracking (ALWAYS check with your doctor, as this could indicate a yeast infection called *Perlache*)	Mycolog ointment (Rx, anti-yeast, anti-inflammatory)	Aquaphor	Bag Balm
	Nystatin cream (Rx) mixed with Aquaphor	Desitin Rapid Relief	Diluted White Vinegar Soak
	Mupirosin (Rx, also protects against infection MRSA)		
	Silvadene Cream 1% (Rx)		
	Elidel (Rx)		
Radiation Dermatitis (redness, scaling, itching)	Biafine (Rx)	Vanicream Moisturizing Skin Cream	7 Cream
	Corticosteroids (Rx)	AmLactin Moisturizing Lotion	White Vinegar soak (see appendix)
	Clobetasol 0.05% (Rx)	Aquaphor	
	Evozac Calming Skin Spray	Osmotics Triceran	
	Lindi Soothing Balm	Aveeno Daily Moisturizing Lotion	
	My Girls Radiation Cream	Nouriva Repair Moisturizing Cream	

Symptom			
Hand-Foot Syndrome	Radx Radiation Therapy		
	Radx Moisture Therapy		
	Alra Therapy Lotion		
	Linacare Intensive Hand Therapy Cream	Vanicream Moisturizing Skin Cream	Skin Free Niaouli Butter Stick
	EvoSkin Palm and Sole Moisturizing Spray	Neutrogena Norwegian Formula Hand Cream	
	EvoSkin Palm and Sole Moisturizing Cream	Neutrogena Norwegian Formula Cracked Heel Moisturizing Treatment	
	Elasto-Gel Glove	Lotil Cream	
	Lindi Soothing Balm	Dr. Scholl's Massaging Gel Insoles	
	Lindi Skin Cooler Roll and Pad	TheraPedic Cooling Insoles	
Hot flashes/burning sensation	Zonalon (Rx)	Avène Thermal Spring Water Gel	Comfrey Root extract oil
	Lindi Skin Cooler Roll and Pad		

	Carrington HydroGauze Wound Dressing	
Deoderant	Alra Non-Metallic Deoderant	Innocent Oils Pure Himilayan Crystal Body Spray
	EvoDeo Deoderant Spray	

Beneficial Skin Care Ingredients

Please note: this list is not exhaustive. Always check in with your doctor before trying any new treatments.

	Hi-Tech	Natural
Moisturizing	Hyaluronic acid: a hydrophilic – i.e. water-attracting – moisturizer. Good for dry skin.	Argan Oil: an ancient remedy now one of the hottest emollients around. High in Vitamin E, it can even be considered cancer-fighting: a study in *Cancer Detection and Prevention* showed that the growth of three types of in vitro human prostate cancer cells was inhibited 48 hours after being treated with the sterols and polyphenols from Argan oil.
	sodium PCA: a hydrating ingredient.	Shea butter: emollient (promotes soothing)
	Sorbitol: a hydrating ingredient.	Avocado: emollient
	Silicone: a hydrating ingredient.	Olive oil: emollient
	Ceramides: emollient.	Aloe: emollient
	Glycerin: A hydrating ingredient	Arnica: emollient
		Chamomile: emollient, relieves redness
		Arnica: emollient
		Honey: a humectant (draws in water)
		Algae extract: hydrating

Soothing	Azelaic acid: calms redness/rosacea	Chamomile: relieves redness
	Sodium sulfacetamide: calms redness/rosacea	Pro-biotics: decreases bacteria that can cause inflammation
	Topical metronidazole: calms redness/rosacea	Colloidal oatmeal: soothes itchiness
	Vitamin K: relieves redness	Argan Oil: nourishes the skin and reduces inflammation
Acne	Salicylic acid: an oil-dissolving acid.	Tea Tree Oil: anti-bacterial, anti-fungal and antiseptic, it heals pimples and decreases irritation
	Topical antibiotics: clean out pores, treat blemishes.	Lavender: antiseptic that also aids in scar reduction
		Willow Bark Extract: a natural form of salicylic acid, it aids in cell turnover and reduces inflammation
		Sulfur: smells bad but is a good cleansing and drying agent
		Argan Oil: regulates oily skin
Dark Spots/ Hyperpigmentation	Vitamin C: An anti-oxidant that reduces redness and dark spots	Green and white teas: anti-oxidant that also helps dark spots
	Hydroquinone: dark spots, brightens skin	Bearberry: skin brightener

	Haloxyl: dark spots, peptide which brightens skin	Licorice: skin brightener
		Argan Oil: aids in fading scars
Protection	Vitamin C: An anti-oxidant that protects against radical damage.	Grapeseed oil: anti-oxidant that reduces radical damage

Dental Health Treatments

Please note: this list is not exhaustive. Always check in with your doctor before trying any new treatments.

Condition	Prescription	Over the Counter	Natural		
Dry Mouth	Optimoist Mouth Spray	Biotene Dry Mouth Fluoride Toothpaste, Oral Rinse and Moisturizing Mouth Spray	Borage Oil		
	Caphasol rinse	Farley's Entertainer's Secret Throat Relief Spray	Drink water often and suck on ice chips (called Cryotherapy)		
	Pilocarpine HCI (Salagen), a drug that stimulates salivary flow	Hard sugarless lemon drops	Humidifier in bedroom at night		
	Prescription toothpaste with higher fluoride content	Oasis Dry Mouth Moisturizing Spray	Natural ice popcicles		
	Amifostine (Ethyol) – protects against the damage of radiation	Sugarless chewing gum with xylitol			
	Cevimeline (Evoxac)	Sensodyne Toothpaste			
		Colgate PreviDent 500 (a high fluoride toothpaste)			

Mouth Sores	Magic Mouthwash (aka Pink Mouthwash, a custom-made mixture of antibiotic, antihistamine, antifungal, steroid and/or antacid). One expert recommends a combination of Lidocaine (to numb the mouth), Benadryl (antihistamine) and Maalox (for sour stomach that can accompany the sores).	Sugar free mints containing xylitol	Deglycyrrhizinated Licorice lozenges (commonly referred to as DGL)
	Gelclair (a muco-adherent)	Biotene Oral Balance	Rinsing with ice water and sucking ice chips
	Palifermin (Kepivance), and IV Medication	Orajel	Baking soda rinse: ½ tsp. Salt, 2 tbs. Baking soda dissolved in 4 cups water.
	Caphosol (a prescription mouthwash)	Maalox, Mylanta, Milk of Magnesia: coating your blisters with these antacids might help.	Coating agents such as kaolin solutions
	Chlorhexidine rinse (Peridex, Perioguard) - apply with a cotton swab to affected areas	Betadine Gargle and Mouthwash	Kamillosan rinse (made from camomile)
	Topical analgesics and anti-inflammatories such as Benzydamine HCI topical rinse	Coating agents such as kaolin solutions (Kaopectate)	Natural ice popcicles
	Topical anesthetic agents (Zylocaine 2-5%, Lidocaine, Benzocaine gels/sprays, or Diclonin hydrochloride. 5-1%).	Zilactin Cold Sore Gel	Rinses made with Rosemary and Thyme

Aluminum hydroxide capsules or suspension	Swab sores with a hydrogen peroxide/saltwater solution: 1 part 3% hydrogen peroxide, 2 parts seawater made of 1 tsp salt in 4 cups of water)	Rinses made with marshmallow leaves
Cellulose agents that form a film over sores confined to a local area (Hydroxypropyl cellulose)		
Pilocarpine HCI (Salagen), a drug that stimulates salivary flow		
Pain relief: Difflam (benzydamine hydrochloride) before meals	Pain relief: topic analgesics, aspirin	
Prostaglandin (PGE) – but not used following HSCT	Ulcerease Anesthetic Mouth Rinse	
Kamillosan	Cepacol Sore Throat Oral Pain Reliever Lozenges	
Sucralfate (brand name Carafate, aluminum salt of sucrose ostasulphate). This creates a surface barrier with cytoprotective effect, meaning it protects cells from damage)	Colgate Orabase B Paste with Benzocaine	
Amifostine (Ethyol) – protects against the damage of radiation	Advil, Tylenol for pain relief	
Zilactin	Rincinol PRN	
	Ambesol	

Cavities		See your dentist; begin fluoride treatment					
Sensitive Teeth							
Tooth loosening in gums		See your dentist					
Jaw stiffening and loss of mobility							
Bleeding mouth and gums							
Osteoradionecrosis (ORN or ONJ)		See your dentist					

Made in the USA
Middletown, DE
02 May 2016